WAR

ON AGING

**DR. PATSI KRAKOFF
ROBERT KRAKOFF**

This book is intended as a reference volume only, not as a medical manual. The information given here is designed to help you make informed decisions about your health. It is not intended as a substitute for any treatment that may have been prescribed by your doctor. If you suspect you have a medical problem, we urge you to seek competent medical help.

The information in this book is meant to supplement, not replace, proper exercise training. All forms of exercise pose some inherent risks. The authors advise readers to take full responsibility for their health and safety and to know their limits. Before practicing exercise, be sure equipment is well-maintained, and do not take risks beyond your level of experience, aptitude, training, and fitness. The exercise and dietary programs in this book are not intended as a substitute for any exercise routine or dietary regimen that may have been prescribed by your doctor. As with all exercise and dietary programs, you should get your doctor's approval before beginning.

Mention of specific companies, organizations, or authorities in this book does not imply endorsement by the authors, nor does mention of specific companies, organizations, or authorities imply that they endorse this book or its authors.

Internet addresses given in this book were accurate at the time of publication.

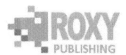

TABLE OF CONTENTS

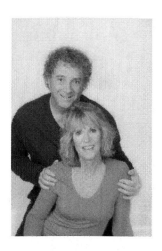

"Age is just a number"

1   The Premise and a Promise

Have you noticed? Today's seniors don't look or act much like "old people."

Seniors are much "younger" these days. And yet, when we reach that age—usually after 50 or 65—we notice there are a lot of different factors affecting our bodies and brains, and we wonder: what should we be doing about it? Or is it too late?

There's not much good advice or any new guidelines to turn to when it comes to learning how to age well. Our grandparents and parents didn't have the same possibilities we do. They just accepted aging and grew older—and usually weaker and sicker—without questioning it.

This is a new era where many seniors over 70 and 80, even 90, are still very active, playing sports, living energetically, and participating fully in ways not expected in previous generations. Some run marathons, do bodybuilding, write books, participate in arts and entertainment, and are even into online dating.

Roughly 10,000 baby boomers turn 65 in the U.S. every day, and more of them are not giving in to old age. Like us, they're fighting back.

Contemporaries and family may tell us we're too old to do this or that, but we're not listening. Sure, we're limited by some physical conditions, but we're also finding ways to work around obstacles and injuries and stay as active as we can, no matter what. We're joining the Senior War on Aging and we're being rewarded physically and mentally.

The New Senior Imperative

We include anyone over the age of 50 as a senior, since the aging process begins to attack us in earnest after that age. The new imperative for anyone over 50 is to exercise. Nothing else will do as much to delay the decaying process and eliminate many of the chronic diseases of old age. While aging is inevitable, decay is not. Our bodies and our brains depend on being active. We, the authors, Dr. Patsi and husband Rob Krakoff, both strongly believe that if you start now, you can stay fit for the rest of your life.

If this sounds impossible, perhaps you aren't aware of some of the awesome medical technologies already in development that will extend lives and health. If we can stay alive long enough to benefit from these incredible advances, we can ameliorate the effects of heart problems, diabetes, cancer, bone loss, vision and hearing loss, dementia, and other common causes of misery in old age.

We'll share some of what's happening in medical technology. For example, nanobots are cell-sized computers that can be injected into the blood stream to take care of dysfunctions and disease. This is not science fiction; already Parkinson's patients are using brain implants.[1]

Hyaluronic acid injections are now available to make joint cartilage more viscous and stem cell implants are being perfected to promote cartilage regeneration. Adult stem cells can be isolated and replicated from your own body fat, then injected back into an area that needs healing or regeneration. Stem cell therapies are being used for joint and tissue injuries, herniated and bulging discs, diabetes, organ

3

damage, autoimmune diseases, neurological diseases, and traumatic brain injuries.

As seniors, we need to stay alive another decade, long enough for these breakthroughs to become available. They will extend our quality of life and there will be other inventions. But the key is to stay alive and well-functioning until some of the chronic diseases of aging are eliminated, which is the point of this book.

According to Ray Kurzweil and Dr. Terry Grossman in *Transcend: Nine Steps to Living Well Forever*, with the mapping of the human genome complete, non-embryonic stem cell therapy, bionic replacement parts, and cloned organs are on track for realization by the early 2020s, and nanotechnology will follow in the 2030s.[2]

For now, the only solution science currently has for seniors to remain healthy is through exercise, good nutrition, medications, and supplements. Exercise can override the body's preprogrammed genetic message to decay.

We are convinced that when it comes to senior fitness, attention to physical, emotional, and mental health can be the fountain of youth. When we exercise and are active we tap into our bodies' reserves, staying youthful and healthy longer.

Unfortunately, however, many seniors have bought into the concept that aging equals decay. They accept that as an inevitable fact, probably because many of them saw their parents and grandparents go through such misery. The idea that we can slow down the aging process, and in some cases, reverse it to avoid chronic illness, seems unrealistic.

Mind Shifts for Old Dogs

We'd like to reverse that mindset and encourage everyone to join the Senior War on Aging, but first, seniors must believe that it is possible to be healthier. A shift in one's mental model is required, and some "old folks" don't shift easily. In fact, since most of us have been practicing our standard health habits for so long, we resist when told we need to change them.

Why do you think so many seniors ignore good advice about exercise and diet? Likely, they're thoroughly entrenched in habits of a lifetime based on incomplete knowledge from medical experts of the past. Today, we know much more about the body and the brain.

We know from brain scans and imaging that you CAN teach old dogs new tricks. But it's like the old joke about how many psychologists it takes to change a light bulb: it takes only one but she must want to change it.

We believe seniors would modify some of their health habits if they knew what leading-edge healthcare specialists know about aging well. Any senior who wants to age better than his parents did can do so by shifting his mental model to what's possible.

Aging Does Not Equal Decay

While exercise and diet are super important, there is first a vital need to cultivate the right attitude from which to operate. From what we see, so many people have bought into the "aging = decay" paradigm that they don't realize what's truly possible for them. Most of us will need to rewire our thinking alongside tactical actions like exercising most days of the week.

Dr. Christiane Northrup makes this point in her excellent book, *Goddesses Never Age:*

> *Ageless living is what you experience when you engage in life without fear that you're going to fall – or fall apart...we need to be more aware of our culture's negative messages about growing older and make a conscious effort to reject them.*[3]

What we believe is critical because it will determine the actions we take. No one can get fit if they don't believe exercise is worth it and that it will pay off. Some people think it's not worth the effort, they're never going to get their figure back or be fit, and what's the point—they're old!

Getting Fit, One Cell at a Time

Exercise is much more than looking young and fit; it's about feeling healthy and happy while we age. It's about being able to be active and enjoy life. It's about delaying the decay on a cellular level.

Our goal is to move fellow seniors out of the old paradigm of experiencing aging like their parents and grandparents did. We want to see everyone up and exercising. We'll show you how to plan the time to exercise, to improve strength, endurance, and flexibility. We'll remind you of the importance of shopping for real food and preparing meals that will make you feel and think "fit for life" as we age.

Rob and I both live an active life and strive to motivate others to get on board and ride the "exercise train" to a longer, wiser, and more fulfilling senior adventure.

Our promise to you is that even if you follow only a few of our suggestions, you will benefit from reading this book—and in ways you don't expect. You will look better, feel better, and your body and brain will put the brakes on the slide into old age and debilitation.

One Proviso

My husband Rob knows a great deal about the body and exercise. He is a superb athlete in tennis, football, and baseball, was on the Navy's Special Services team as a boxer, played AAU basketball, and rode in mountain bike rallies from San Diego to Las Vegas. Not everyone can relate to his experiences, so what he does and says may not appeal to you for your own fitness program.

In other words, just because we often spend two or three hours a day exercising doesn't mean you should. Only a few years ago, the thought of ten minutes in the gym seemed to me like a climb up Mt. Everest. Some days it still does, but I use mental tricks to get going. Everyone has to start at their own level and work up as they can.

We're addressing all levels of conditions, including how to exercise without getting or exacerbating an injury. We invite you to examine excuses, weed out false or outdated beliefs, and decide how, when, and where to get started.

Not being an accomplished professional-level athlete myself, I'm writing from the other perspective—from a woman's view, but also as someone who hasn't trained for sports over a lifetime.

I was that girl who hits the gym in spurts. My idea of a power walk was covering all three floors of Nordstrom's with a credit card in hand.

Today, at age 73, I'm better off than I admit. Working out and playing sports grows on a person, as it did for me. If you give it a good try and sustain it over a period of time, you will become a fit person, no matter your age or the shape you're in now.

Male or female, all seniors can fight decay and aging, no matter their conditions. Everyone has a right to live long, strong, and enjoy life. It's worth it. You're worth it.

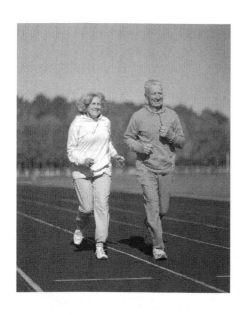

2   There's a War Going On

ROB SAYS

In many ways, becoming a senior is like fighting a losing battle, but it's a fight well worth engaging in. Nobody gets out alive, but sometimes you need to fight a little longer, harder, and persistently. Never give up until it's time to go. And even then, don't stop fighting, because in a few more years we will have more life-saving options available to us.

That's what I told our friend Julie. She was getting a wakeup call. She was angry and felt slighted that age was catching up with her. The fact was, her body was changing. Not as much on the outside as on the inside.

"Julie, I hate to tell you this because you look so healthy and gorgeous. You need to follow up with the doctor on your symptoms and health indicators. I know you don't want to hear this, but you're getting older.

"Realizing you're getting older and your body is aging is hard to accept, especially if you've always practiced healthy habits. Any time a senior gets sick, the whole system is unbalanced and affected. Any illness or injury is harder to recover from, and usually leaves debris."

A few days later, Julie told me that understanding that aging is like a war made her feel more energized. She felt ready to engage, having passed through anger and denial. She could muster up an action plan, get more information from her doctor, and use her energy to draw up a combat program.

If that meant more exercise, or a change in activities, diet, and supplements, she was ready to do what it would take. She told me she'd follow her doctor's advice and start taking red yeast rice, vitamin E, and other supplements to lower her cholesterol. After three or four months, she'd get retested. She told me, "I'll take a prescription medication if I have to at that point."

If you face each day knowing you are going to be challenged because your body is aging, you can enlist your reserves and become willing to go the extra mile with a smile.

As seniors, we're at war, a war on aging, and we aren't going to back down.

Two Key Issues

No matter our age or condition, there are two things we seniors can pay attention to right way if we want to be successful in the war against premature decay.

1. Prevention

What can we do to prevent illnesses and conditions from taking hold in our bodies? What about diet, supplements, and pollutants that cause possible toxic reactions? We need to become better informed about preventing illness and injuries. We can ask our doctors, but sometimes they have been trained to focus more on curing diseases after the fact. It's up to us as seniors to educate ourselves through books, health sites, organizations, and gyms that promote healthy lifestyles. If your doctor isn't sure about current prevention measures, find a healthcare professional who is.

2. Early Detection

The second thing we can do as healthy seniors is to monitor early signs of possible dysfunction. Without being paranoid, we can request regular checks for cancer, diabetes, heart conditions, memory loss, and a host of common conditions of aging. Early detection will up the odds in favor of survival. Ask your doctor what's recommended.

Doctors who stay abreast of current trends already know about these things. Yet Patsi and I have found that not all medical practitioners are experienced enough regarding exercise and fitness levels for older people. This could stem from the fact that they themselves don't exercise or play sports, or they may be too young to appreciate what is possible for seniors.

And, quite frankly, I've found that some doctors just don't think older people are going to go to a gym and work out. They underestimate us! Don't let your doctor assume you are ready for the rocking chair. While one should always check with a physician before beginning any exercise activity, it's also good to consult with a doctor who is knowledgeable about sports and exercise for active seniors.

Julie's situation is common among individuals who already practice sports and healthy habits and have done so for most of their lives. Signs of aging often come gradually, gently, and unobtrusively: a few skin changes, slower reaction time, less balance, gradual weight gain, and less energy. Occasionally we can't remember a name as quickly as before. But sometimes, as in Julie's case, symptoms strike in groups and suddenly.

When Julie's cholesterol levels rose from 215 to 285, her doctor recommended Lipitor, a statin drug with side effects. Her lab report also showed thyroid levels requiring medication. And, she was dealing with a ringing in her ears.

For the first time in her life, Julie felt like she was losing control of her health. And because of her strong personality traits, this wasn't something she found easy to just "breathe into."

I can totally relate to this feeling. My own feelings of helplessness over health occurred when I reached the age range when my first-degree family members died (50-60). You may feel as if you have reached your own point of no return.

No Way Out?

The hard truth is that we are genetically programmed to age, to self-destruct. We possess an outdated genetic program that wants us to die young. Even so, we can work out, watch what we eat, avoid sugars and trans fats, and extend life into the 80s, the 90s and beyond.

Sure, we know that death will get us in the end. Worse, illness and disability will make living miserable for some of us before we finally croak.

From the end of our child-bearing years, and even before, our cells start to decay. We enjoy optimal health for a relatively short time; then, gradually, the struggle begins and deterioration sets in.

But Wait! What If...

What if you drank a few cups of green tea, ate five servings of fruits and vegetables, exercised at least 30 minutes to elevate your heart rate, ate some fish, took some recommended nutritional supplements, spent some quality time with friends, and got eight hours of good sleep? Then you probably would have aged very little today.

If we're going to take charge and advocate for our bodies' health, we need education. This may mean going beyond Internet health sites. In our appendixes, we recommend a few books with innovative research on exercise, nutrition, and longevity issues.

My Perspective as a Psychologist

When Rob decided to write this book on senior fitness, I jumped on board as quickly as a bunny rabbit. There are only a few things I know well enough to write about with passion. Staying alive and active is a driving force in my life.

As a psychologist, I hear a lot about the challenges of growing older. Some seniors have adopted the *BMW* attitude: bitching, moaning, and whining all the way.

Other seniors approach the aging process differently. They are happy to finally be working at something they love in their "third age," whether they're only partially retired or have started a new project or rekindled a favorite hobby.

As we age, we have the liberty to carve out a niche of old interests we never had time for when we were working. I know former schoolteachers who take up dancing, bankers who grow orchids, and people who've turned into actors, singers, writers, computer nerds, photographers, and musicians—no matter their previous careers.

Unfortunately, many of us don't have the physical strength to do what we used to do. And it's no wonder after a lifetime of going to an office, sitting on our butts, and eating junk food. Worse, even our previously sharp brains fail us at times, giving us fears about creeping dementia and Alzheimer's.

Most women I know share that they'd love to get back into exercising or a sport, but each time they try, they're faced with failure, soreness, injuries, boredom, or lack of confidence in themselves. Who wants to spend time with that? No one does.

It's easy to give in to "I'm just getting older so what's the use?" thinking. Or, you can just say "no" to that way of thinking. "*Just do it*" would be smarter… but then, you'd have to actually *do* it, wouldn't you?

Why Not "Just Do It"?

Here's the hard truth, it's really "*just do it or die!*" If we don't exercise, we may not die right away; we may live a long time but in unhealthy ways. Without attention to health, exercise, and nutrition, it's almost certain that we'll end up facing some nasty conditions and diseases as we age.

Experts say seniors can eliminate about 50 to 70 percent of common diseases of aging by exercising.[1] We think so too.

Our Invitation to Join the War on Aging

Doctors know about how exercise is vital to healthy seniors, but I think many give up on their patients. They are well-trained to respond to disease or injuries. Few know how to motivate people to adopt basic steps for prevention. The doctors' dilemma is that they know so much that can help patients remain healthy, but don't know how to get them to make the necessary changes. They see too many seniors who are "non-compliant" with their doctors' recommendations. So, even though they know exercise is key to longevity, they aren't equipped to make sure senior patients follow through. It's not enough to simply tell seniors they need to exercise.

Rob and I ask you to join us in the Senior War on Aging. We can do a lot for ourselves to ensure our "golden years" are enjoyable. We must keep the body's programmed decay to a bare minimum.

The right mindset must come first, a learner's mindset. You are largely in charge of your health, and hopefully, with the guidance of a good physician, you can decide how you will shift to a healthier lifestyle, one that is appropriate for your fitness level.

Two Obstacles

If you want to stay healthy and live an active, satisfying life, exercise is never "one and done." The seniors we see today looking and moving younger than their years have adopted a consistent exercise habit. The ones winning the war on aging have confronted two difficult obstacles:

1. Daily exercise

"What? I have to start exercising every day???"

You do, yes. Well, only if you want to lessen the chance of getting sick, of being miserable, of having physical and mental limitations, and of dying prematurely from preventable diseases.

Get out there and move your feet. You will have to sweat. Whatever you're doing now is good, but probably not enough. Start where you are, according to your fitness level, and work up to the levels that can help extend your life and health.

2. Daily Exercise—Every Day

Not only do we need to start exercising every day, but we must keep on doing it, every day. I must repeat myself here: If you want to have a longer life with less pain and more vitality, you need to start exercising almost every day, and do it forever.

There's no end where you sit down and say, "There, I'm fit." Aim for six days a week, mixing up different kinds of exercises and activities.

To me, that's not a bad deal at all. But I didn't always feel that way, and I haven't been rigorously strict about it. After a lot of reading on the new science of aging well, I've shifted my haphazard, "good enough" exercise habits.

The research is clear: all the evidence points to a much bigger role for exercise if seniors want to age well, extend life and health spans, and avoid the many chronic debilitations of getting old.

Just like brushing teeth is a habit we don't have to think about, so should be exercise. We need to repeatedly exercise over a long period to get all the great health and longevity benefits. Some benefits we can see right away, and some we might never see, but they are there, keeping us alive and healthy.

It's always harder to do things when we don't see awesome results right away, isn't it? But then, we've brushed our teeth for how many years now? Remember, exercise most days of the week will build up the immune system, regulate the heart muscle, build new brain cells, strengthen joints and bones, and prevent a lot of misery that comes with age.

Each time we exercise, the muscles unleash a cascade of chemicals on a cellular level, sending growth signals. We can't see or feel them but our body, brain, muscles, and every cell in our body become an accomplice to health and longevity.

If Not Now, When?

It's never too late to start. As senior women, we've started many different "lives" and careers and had many different roles. So, exercising, as part of the daily habit of growing older, will in some ways be easy for us to do.

21

It's much easier to exercise at 70 if we've been doing it from the age of 50 or 60. Starting early will build a foundation of muscle strength and flexibility that we'll need if we want to stay injury- and disease-free. Whatever your age, remember to start exercising at a level that's comfortable, and build up gradually to avoid injuries.

Now, we know many seniors who are already very active with stuff—hobbies, walking, yoga, and water aerobics. Here's the thing, though. A leisurely stroll around the block or a dip in the pool isn't going to spark life-extension and disease-prevention benefits of a true exercise program.

Don't waste time and energy with inadequate efforts. We recommend 30 minutes of cardiovascular activity four to five days a week with an elevated heart rate (think *sweat*). AND, two to three days a week lifting weights or doing weight-bearing activities to build strength, balance, and flexibility. That's an end goal, not a starting-out point.

Even if you start with 10 or 20 minutes three days a week, you're doing untold good for your body and brain. The idea is to start at your appropriate fitness level and work up to 30 or even 45 minutes of cardio and two to three days of strength training, including a variety of movements and sports for fun.

We don't think this amount is too much, and we're not alone here either. Many scientists, fitness experts, and medical doctors also recommend this level of activity for seniors.

Perhaps the biggest obstacle to exercising is that "muscle" between the ears: the brain. To get healthy and live longer, we'll have to get smart and outsmart our "stinking thinking."

There are many false beliefs people buy into: not enough time, it's too late for me to get fit, I've got too many aches and pains, what's the use?

Look, we've all used these and other excuses to not exercise. I sometimes joke I've got a PhD in making excuses.

However you look at it, none of us have ever been this old before, or faced as many brutal challenges as the aging process presents. Did you have any idea getting old would happen to you and be so damned hard? So far, the only thing that's saved us from *BMW* (bitching, moaning, and whining) is exercise. It's saved my life, saved my body, and saved my mind from depression more than once.

My Story

Although my husband's been a lifelong jock, I haven't. I've been fairly active but sucked at sports. As a child, I was extremely nearsighted, couldn't see a baseball, and never got picked for teams. I had long limbs and no muscle definition. If I gained weight it was all belly fat. I looked like a tomato held up by two toothpicks.

Each time I'd join a gym, the trainer did his fitness evaluations, and I was always in the below-average range. But at some point, all that changed.

How I ended up as a model in Paris in the 1970s is another story, but it was then that I became hooked on looking good. When I first started working out, I struggled with self-discipline, weight, and balancing good nutrition with partying and night life.

Around my 40th birthday I had an epiphany. Maybe it was all that existentialism in Paris, but I began thinking there was more to life. Maybe I was missing something important. I quit drinking, partying, smoking, and took up exercising with a personal trainer. I went back to school, studied psychology, and got my doctorate, and a few decades have slipped by since then.

That is not to say I've been a well-disciplined exerciser and fitness buff for all that time. No, rather, I rode the roller coaster like many women: one day up, another down, and around and around it all goes.

Until one day I realized I had made a great deal of progress despite it all. Evidently, over the course of many years, I had accumulated more healthy days than not.

Somewhere down the road, I grew healthy habits, got rid of a few negative ones, and it got easier. I now think of myself as a "healthy person;" it's part of who I am. It doesn't feel good to not act healthy. I feel bad when I'm engaging in laziness, junk food, and excuses.

I must warn you, it took me a lot of time and work to get this way. That doesn't mean it will take you a long time. I hope not. But even if it does, it's worth it.

Starting in my sixties, some people remarked how young and fit I looked. Curious about their comments, I had some measurements taken at the gym for strength and flexibility.

And I couldn't believe it. At some point, after off-and-on gym and sports regimens, I passed over into the "excellent physical condition" range. I don't think I got that much more fit, but women my age, to whom they compare, were getting increasingly unfit. All I had to do was keep going to the gym, eat a healthy diet, and not die, and eventually I got in the range of excellent.

So, if you stay at it long enough, you will get fit. Oh, and you must stay alive also. So many people our age don't do that, and that's sad. I must disagree when they say, "Living well is the best revenge."

Quite frankly, just staying alive is good enough for me.

No matter your current state, you can increase your fitness level. Very few of us seniors are going to achieve bodybuilder status; that's not the objective. Like Rob, I believe that most of us don't exercise as much as necessary to get the life-prolonging cellular benefits. To me, that's the real goal: improved cellular health that will ensure a better, longer, and "younger" old-age.

Everyone's different and has different reasons for staying healthy. For me, it has to do with everyone in my family dying young (50s and 60s)—from heart disease, cancers, and alcoholism. I don't want my life to be cut short now, because I'm having too much fun and enjoying myself more each year.

I don't want to become debilitated either. It's hard enough to not be able to do everything we could when we were young, but I still like to carry my own groceries, open jars, shop for hours, play tennis, and dance. Especially tap dancing. That always makes me happy.

You can't live forever, granted, but you can try to stay strong and active for as long as possible.

Bonus Gifts for Our Readers

10 Mistakes Healthy Seniors Make
(...and their consequences in 5-10 years)

You may think you're doing okay because you're still healthy. The habits you have today will determine if you thrive as a senior... or barely survive.

For this report and other special gifts to our readers, visit our private page:

www.seniorfitness4life.com/thanks-enlisting-war-aging/

27

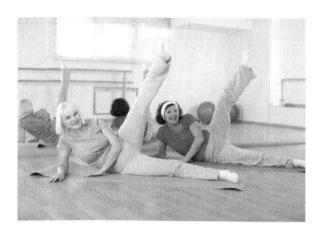

3   A New Age for Seniors

In the past 100 years, medical science has managed to extend our lifespan from the early 40s to our late 70s and early 80s. In Japan, life expectancy is already into the 80s. From a technology standpoint, the next 10 years will equal the past 100 in scientific advancements and discoveries. Biomedical advances, public health initiatives, and social changes will further reduce mortality and increase longevity.

The Future of Healthcare

Did you know that scientists are already working on perfecting nanobots? These cell-sized robots can be injected into your body to seek and destroy harmful pathogens, genetic dysfunctions, and cancer cells.

Nanobots could also be used to deliver RNA interference which turns off genes such as the fat insulin receptor, thereby eliminating diabetes and obesity.

The Extension of Our Health Spans

A longer lifespan isn't necessarily a good thing. How valuable is a longer life if we simply increase the number of years we're alive? We suggest aiming for longer "health spans." The goal is to live longer AND extend the number of years we are healthy and active.

How to spend those extra years is in our control to some extent. Will we live our remaining senior years in active, productive, fulfilling endeavors, or will our golden years be dull, overshadowed by declining health, loss of memory, and lingering illness?

Science is most likely going to figure this all out one day and provide some solutions for aging: better sensory functioning and digestion, better organs, better joints and replacements, and radical treatments of diseases. That makes our quality of life an even greater concern if we want to thrive, not just survive.

Our ideas are based on far more than just the combined personal experiences of a former professional athlete and a non-athletic motivational psychologist. Our evidence comes from:

1. **Science:** Every day, new studies reveal the benefits of exercise and diet—particularly for

seniors who can prevent or delay the onset of disabilities and diseases and increase their longevity. Some experts say that 50 percent of so-called "diseases of aging" can be prevented or eliminated altogether by exercise. Longevity research points to exercise as both prevention and a cure for physical and mental health: decreased risk of heart disease, obesity, cancer, diabetes, and osteoporosis, as well as dementia and Alzheimer's.

2. **Evolutionary biology:** Our genetics haven't changed much since we were running, hunting, and gathering food on the savannas of Africa. Humans began to evolve rapidly with the use of language, tools, and social cooperation about 10,000 years ago. In only the last 100 years, humans have doubled their average lifespan, but we still have the same basic genetic makeup as when we were living in primitive tribes. Our genetic code tells our body to grow when we move, and to decay when we don't. But even though aging is inevitable, decay is not. We don't have to act our age and we certainly do not have to feel old. To stave off decay we need to do something physical nearly every day. While

we can't stop aging, we can delay and stop the deterioration.

ROB SAYS

Aging is a stern taskmaster. There are constant daily reminders of our advancing years. We have been fortunate enough to have lived through wars, diseases, nasty fast foods, and reality TV. Those of us who have reached our 60s, 70s and 80s are the true survivors. According to the Centers for Disease Control and Prevention, the average life expectancy for American males is 78.8 years. (I must write fast, as my expiration date is approaching.)

As the final battle nears, I do not ascribe to minimums, stopgaps, or quick fixes. Nor do I believe in pseudo-scientific pills, potions, injections, or other life-extending placebos. The only life-extending "pill" known to science is vigorous exercise. Perhaps in the future, nanotechnology, replacement parts, or any number of biotech discoveries will extend life. But the chance of that occurring in my lifetime—unless I can stay alive and healthy enough for another 10 to 20 years— is getting slim.

PATSI SAYS

Every woman faces her own challenges with aging. While men struggle with their diminishing muscles, strength, and hair, we women are the ones who are expected to maintain a degree of beauty, familial wisdom, and serenity throughout life.

Some senior women rush to cosmetic surgeons, dermatologists, spas, and fat farms. There's no doubt that surgery can improve looks, but what good is it if inside you are rotting? Do we really want to look fabulous but not be able to play with the grandkids or take walks with friends?

Senior women must decide how they are going to age well. We are accustomed to wanting it all. Some women finally admit they can't do everything, and some even say, "To hell with it all!"

The real enemy isn't wrinkles or even aging; it's being sedentary. The fountain of youth can't be purchased. It's free. Getting healthy means going back to our roots, to doing what our body is designed for. We were born to run, jump, and play. Not moving our bodies is what is unnatural.

Not everyone wants a generalized approach to fitness. Some want to focus on regaining lost flexibility or upper body or leg strength, some want to lose weight, and some simply want to cut to the chase and learn the deeper secrets of longevity.

Some Simple Steps to Start

What does it mean to live a healthy senior life? Let's get started with a few simple things everyone can do to start living more healthfully.

1. Eat Organic Food

This includes eating whole foods such as real butter, whole grains instead of refined grains, fresh fruits, vegetables, and beans to provide fiber and vitamins. We need to eat fish, low-fat meats, and skinless chicken cooked with healthy, natural spices. We can learn to stay away from fried foods, processed foods, and chemical additives. Baking, poaching, and slow cooking methods avoid the high-heat adulteration of fats that may be dangerous to our cellular metabolism. The world is full of fresh berries and fruit that our bodies need to stay alive and fight diseases and aging.

2. Get Some Sunshine

Exposure to sunlight increases the release of the serotonin hormone in your brain. Exposure to the ultraviolet B in the sun's rays causes a person's skin to create vitamin D, which plays a big role in bone health. Moderate amounts of sunlight have cancer preventive benefits for colon cancer, Hodgkin's lymphoma, ovarian cancer, pancreatic cancer, and prostate cancer.

According to the World Health Organization, getting anywhere from 5 to 15 minutes of sunlight on your arms, hands, and face two to three times a week is enough to enjoy the vitamin D-boosting benefits of the sun. Note that the sun must actually penetrate the skin—wearing sunscreen or clothing won't result in vitamin D production—so I recommend getting sun early in the day or later in the afternoon to avoid sunburn and skin cancer.

3. Switch to Natural Cleaning Products

Somewhere in the 1950s some marketing genius decided to create powerful household cleaning products to make domestic life easier. Today the modern home is loaded with toxic polluting substances caused by these same commercial cleaning products. One in three people suffers from allergies, asthma, sinusitis, or bronchitis directly related to these household cleaning chemicals. Some chemical ingredients don't even have to be listed on labels. For example, the word "fragrance" is allowed instead of naming the actual chemicals used in the product. Some of these have not been tested or have had negative side effects.

As wise seniors, we don't have to succumb to the pitfalls of modern marketing and the ploys of industry lobbyists. There are many inexpensive, easy-to-use, natural alternatives which can safely be used in place of commercially-branded products. Here is a list of common, environmentally safe products which can be used alone or in combination for a variety of household applications.

- Baking Soda – cleans, deodorizes, softens water, scours.
- Soap – unscented soap in liquid form, flakes, powders, or bars is biodegradable and will clean just about anything. Avoid using soaps which contain petroleum distillates or any soap marked "antibacterial," as the triclosan contained therein is a known carcinogen.
- Lemon – one of the strongest food acids, effective against most household bacteria.
- Borax (sodium borate) -- cleans, deodorizes, disinfects, softens water, and cleans wallpaper, painted walls, and floors.
- White Vinegar – cuts grease, removes mildew, odors, some stains, and wax build-up.
- Washing Soda – or sal soda, is sodium carbonate decahydrate, a mineral. Washing soda cuts grease, removes stains, softens water, cleans walls, tile, sinks, and tubs. Use care, as washing soda can irritate mucous membranes. Do not use on aluminum.

- Isopropyl Alcohol – is an excellent disinfectant. (It has been suggested to replace this with ethanol or 100 proof alcohol in solution with water. There is some indication that isopropyl alcohol buildup contributes to illness in the body.)
- Cornstarch – can be used to clean windows, polish furniture, shampoo carpets and rugs.
- Citrus Solvent – cleans paint brushes, oil and grease, some stains. (Citrus solvent may cause skin, lung, or eye irritations for people with multiple chemical sensitivities.)

4. **Stop Smoking**

Knowing that we're all aware of the dangers of smoking, do we need to say more? Seniors who still smoke are highly dependent on nicotine and need to rewire their addiction. Exercise is the best method of altering the neural pathways while creating an alternative reward for nicotine. The dopamine and endorphin highs from exercise can help curb the dangerous and debilitating addictions of smoking.

It is never too late to change and the health benefits are almost immediate. Ex-smokers report they taste and smell things more vibrantly, have reduced risk of heart attacks and cancer, fewer respiratory problems, improved circulation, can exercise more, feel more energetic, and they most certainly will live longer.

5. Limit Alcohol Intake

Aging lowers the body's tolerance for alcohol. Older adults generally experience the effects of alcohol more quickly than when they were younger. This puts seniors at higher risk for falls, auto accidents, and other unintentional injuries from drinking. Many prescription and over-the-counter medications, as well as herbal remedies, can be dangerous or even deadly when mixed with alcohol.

Yes, there are health benefits from moderate daily drinking. But don't use that as an excuse to drink more than is recommended.

Heavy drinking will make all the common problems of aging worse, including not remembering how many drinks we've already had, and what medications we've taken. Perhaps the only good thing about it is we won't remember where we put our keys and parked the car, thus lowering our chances of a DUI. And, even if alcohol helps us to have a good time, what good is it if we can't remember it the next day?

Seniors these days are better informed about health and aging than our parents ever were. Many of us are already taking advantage of advanced medical devices and technologies that will keep us alive and active well into our 80s, 90s, and beyond.

And yet, we can't count on artificial means to solve all our health challenges. We are responsible for taking good care of our bodies and minds. All the inventions of science to prolong life won't work well in a poorly-maintained physique.

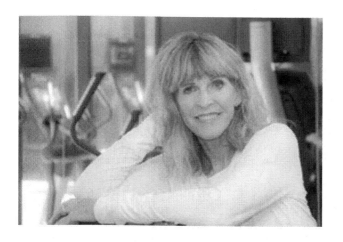

4   Older But Not Aging

Growing older isn't the same thing as aging. Aging is a process that has as its sole purpose the deterioration of health and our ultimate demise. We don't grow old and age at the same rates.

The problem with seniors who give up-- because they're just going to die anyway--is this: more than likely they will *get old and live*. Because of today's advanced healthcare, we will live a long time whether we like it or not. How we live as we age is our choice; we have more control over the aging process than we realize. The question is, are we up for it? Because we are responsible for the quality of our life. And if we want an active, healthy *seniorhood*, we're going to have to work for it. That's why we call this the Senior War on Aging.

As we age, we can lose five to seven pounds of muscle mass every ten years starting in our 30s, and more as we approach our 50s. We also gain about fifteen pounds over the same period. We are genetically programmed to age once we've passed the child-bearing years. Our cells are either growing or decaying, depending on the message we send them. Exercise tells cells to grow. This is reversed with sedentary habits.

Why We Age

The theory as to why we age for years has been, "Aging is nothing more than the buildup of genetic and cellular errors." Noteworthy geneticists, gerontologists, and healthcare practitioners have generally accepted this shared mutational theory as to why we age.

We have been warned of all the detrimental environmental conditions that are getting worse every year. Many of the pollutants that cause DNA errors could be eliminated or avoided. Smoking, obesity, inactivity, alcoholism, stress, and sleep deprivation all contribute to DNA errors.

Our cells have reasonably good repair mechanisms in place. But we'll need more than that.

There is now more research into cellular aging that can help us fight this war.

New discoveries by longevity scientists reveal more causes of aging: some errors in our mitochondrial DNA are due to oxidative stress and more directly related to the food we eat, the water we drink, and the air we breathe. The cells react by triggering inflammation.

Recently, at the University of Tsukuba in Tokyo, Professor Hayashi and his team made a discovery while in the process of addressing some controversial issues surrounding the popular theory of aging alluded to above.

The mitochondrial theory of aging proposes that age-associated mitochondrial defects are caused by the accumulation of toxins in DNA. Abnormal mitochondrial function is one of the hallmarks of aging in many species, including humans. The mitochondrion is the powerhouse of the cell, producing energy in a process called cellular respiration. Damage to the mitochondrial DNA results in mutations in the DNA sequence, and the accumulation of these changes is associated with age-related diseases, reduced lifespan, and early onset of age-related weight gain, hair loss and greying, curvature of the spine, and osteoporosis.

There is, however, conflicting evidence that has raised doubts about this theory. The Tsukuba team performed some compelling research and proposed that age-associated mitochondrial defects are not controlled by the accumulation of mutations in the DNA but by another form of genetic regulation: epigenetic regulation. The research, published in Nature Publishing Group's journal , proposes that epigenetic regulation may be responsible for the age-associated effects seen in the mitochondria.[1]

Epigenetic regulation refers to changes, such as the addition of chemical structures or proteins, which alter the physical structure of the DNA, resulting in genes turning on or off. Unlike mutations, these changes do not affect the DNA sequence itself.

Epigenetic regulation describes anything other than DNA sequence that influences the development of an organism, while mitochondrial theory represents any form of DNA genetic regulation. While aging is determined by our genes, our genes are turned on or off by epigenetic regulation, and subject to environmental influences including nutrition, exercise, and lifestyle choices.

Other research into the causes of aging point to the telomeres, located at the end points of our chromosomes. They become shorter with age, thereby causing faulty DNA replications when cells reproduce. An important enzyme, telomerase, is being studied to prevent or slow down telomere decay.

The important thing to understand is that these studies reveal that, while aging is inevitable, the rate of aging is not. It is now understood that what we put into our bodies and how we use our bodies contributes much more to longevity than inherited genes. The mere fact that our parents lived a long time or died early doesn't mean we will. Lifestyle and health habits are what age us or preserve us. In fact, to put a spin on another aging cliché, you are seldom *as old as you feel*.

As we age, the years pass in rapid succession, and then one day we wake up as a senior, faced with things we've never had to face. I was typical: I experienced the elation of an active and healthy youth, completed an education, labored in a career, raised a family, and now find myself well beyond the age of retirement. It all happened so fast. During a busy life—the life that just sprinted past—maybe you had little or no time for fitness. Is your next step directly into the rocking chair? No, I don't think you want that. Too boring. What will you do? I implore you to not give up. Fight back. Because the war is on. We are all soldiers in the battle to reverse the aging process.

PATSI SAYS

I'm a long-time practitioner of the revered art of denial. I don't lie about my age; I simply don't believe it.

For so long, I've looked younger than my age, acted younger (immature, that is), and dressed youthfully, that I thought "it" wouldn't really happen to me. I avoided talking about "it" or using the "O" word. I wouldn't even make those clichéd senior jokes.

Because everyone in my immediate family died young (50s and 60s), I don't have familiarity with the aging process. With dying, yes; with cancer, yes; I know people die. But growing old and living well as an older person—well, I have no experience seeing others live into their 70s, 80s and 90s. I guess I never thought I'd be around that long.

It turns out longevity experts got it wrong. Instead of life expectancy being determined 90 percent by genes and 10 percent by lifestyle; it's the other way around. If your parents lived into their 90s, you've been blessed with good genetics, so lucky you. But what determines longevity is what you do with the genes you've got—in other words, your lifestyle and health habits.

46

My former reaction to aging had been to act as if it weren't happening. Total denial. I can't do that any longer. Both my looks and body have changed. I get harsh reality signals from the mirror, the tennis courts, and the doctors' offices.

Inactive men and women over age 30 slowly lose muscle tissue every year. At about age 50, this loss of muscle (and strength and endurance) starts happening faster. And after age 65, it accelerates even more. Scientists have a name for muscle loss: sarcopenia. It is from the Greek, meaning "poverty of flesh." It is what we see in frail, elderly people who are bent over from a combination of osteoporosis and low muscle mass, the wasting away of both bone and muscle tissue.

> *If you don't send any signals to grow, decay will win, but even a modest signal to grow—a decent workout, even a good, stiff walk—will drown out the noise. Thing is, you need to do something every day to tell your body it's springtime. ...you have to work at it every day.* ~ Dr. Henry S. Lodge, coauthor of *Younger Next Year: Live Strong, Fit, and Sexy - Until You're 80 and Beyond*[2]

The good news is that the exercise and eating program we recommend is mostly common sense, simple, and fun, with some work—but we try to make that work more like play.

While it's never too late to start exercising, the earlier we begin and the more consistent we are, the greater the long-term rewards. Having an active lifestyle at any age is an investment in your present and future well-being.

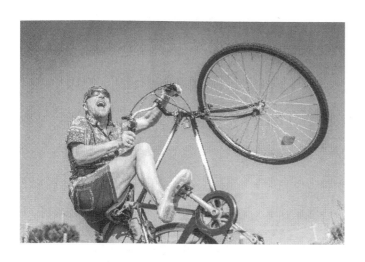

5   Back in the Day...

It seems to me that growing up as I did in the 1940s and 1950s, we never heard of ADD, ADHD, COPD, hepatitis, autism, or bipolar disorders. In the 1940s, people died from heart attacks, influenza, tuberculosis, cholera, malaria, and polio, plus coal miners died from black lung disease. Cancers and heart disease were almost always fatal. And wow, I laughed at the term "anxiety" the first time I heard it described as a medical condition.

While cancers have always been with us, we really didn't hear much about them until the mid-

1970s. That's when our environment began to pummel us with:

- Dramatic increases in processed foods as a major portion of diet

- The switch to diets with a too-high concentration of omega-6 fatty acids and vegetable oils

- Exposure to thousands of industrial toxins never seen in the history of mankind, deregulated by our government, and released into the environment by the ton

- Mass use of known carcinogens such as fluoride in the public water supply

- Explosion of cigarette smoking in society during and after World War II

If that's not scary enough, our bodies and brains are increasingly assaulted by radiation from cell phones and Wi-Fi emissions. The United Nations reports more people have cell phones worldwide than they do access to toilets.[1] We don't yet know the consequences of all this to our health and well-being, at least not on a cellular level.

PATSI SAYS

Rob and I are still young—that is, for our ages! We look and feel strong and can participate in a lot of different activities. And yet, despite our vigorous sports and gym routines, there are some things we avoid because of our individual conditions.

Everyone has them—"conditions": those chronic aches, pains, injuries, or diseases that aren't going to be cured but can be managed. We believe that exercise is probably our best bet for managing these, and feel strongly that exercise will prevent us from getting even more of those annoying old-age conditions.

Sure, one day we'll drop dead like everyone else, but until then we aim to enjoy as many activities as we want. Those, however, may not include trekking in mountains, skydiving, or pole dancing.

Rob's knees have no cartilage left, but he refuses to get replacements as long as he can still play tennis. After his serious heart attack in 2004, he had five stents inserted to keep his arteries open, and now has only about 40 percent heart efficiency. He has a defibrillator implanted in his chest to keep his ticker ticking. Despite that, nothing seems to prevent him from engaging in intense cardiovascular exercise and weightlifting, even though the physicians aren't quite sure how he does it. (Nor do they all agree that he should be doing high levels!)

I've been relatively fortunate as far as my body and joints go. (I guess not doing much in the first half of my life saved me from wearing out joints!) Even so, in 2004, I experienced excruciating lower back and sciatic pain. Two years later, I had successful back surgery with an artificial bone graft and titanium pins inserted at level L4-L5.

I had muscle tear and rotator cuff damage to my right shoulder from tennis and opted for arthroscopic surgery this year. I'm still working out and doing physical therapy to recover, but I hear that after age 70 healing is slow.

My spinal column continues to degenerate and I've lost two inches in height. It aches all the time *except* while playing tennis, thanks to endorphins. My physical exercise includes stretching for decompressing the vertebrae, Pilates to strengthen small muscles and joints, and weightlifting with a trainer to prevent injury. The good news is that my bone density is in the normal range. At one time, tests showed osteopenia, but that's disappeared thanks to my weight-bearing exercises.

Everyone must decide for themselves about surgery, pain, and quality of daily life activities. Here are the most common conditions that require special attention for seniors when it comes to exercise and fitness:

1. Osteoporosis
2. Arthritis
3. Back Pain
4. Injuries (many due to falls)
5. Surgeries

And if those weren't enough...eyes, digestive problems, and sleep quality.

Eyes

We sometimes don't even notice vision problems because changes come on very slowly. It's always better and easier to get treatment early, before problems become magnified.

One area of miraculous medical progress is in ophthalmology. It's becoming common to replace the lens of the eye, for example for cataracts, with a very high success rate. Many seniors have had their vision restored with laser procedures, and statistical results are very favorable.

The key to eye health is to have regular eye exams, even if you believe your vision is fine. You want to avoid letting your eyes deteriorate because you didn't notice any problems, or ignored the signs and symptoms.

Digestive Problems

Let's be honest, who doesn't fart? While it's still socially unacceptable, it's common among seniors and a real problem for many. We don't want to be around others when we're having bouts. Worse still are problems of cramping, diarrhea, constipation, bloating, and burping. Did I forget the dreaded anal leakage?

What has this got to do with fitness and longevity? Well, who wants to go to the gym or do sit-ups or even be around others when we're not sure what noises, smells, or underwear glitches we might have?

This can seriously affect one's social life, as you can imagine! And there is a lot of evidence that a good social life is crucial for longevity.

Sorry to be so graphic about this, but I'm just trying to bring up all the obstacles that will likely get in the way of engaging in a healthy exercise program. Even if you haven't had these conditions yet, you might. Let's confront the reality like grown-ups.

Alternatives

- See your doctor if digestion is a regular problem; get all the tests (colonoscopy, endoscopy), diet recommendations, medications, or suggested remedies.

- Check out some of the common-sense guidelines found online at medical sites like WebMD, Amazon books, and natural health resources.
- Avoid food your system doesn't do well with.
- Remember that walking and exercise help regularity.
- Eat more high-fiber fruits and veggies, but be aware that sometimes they contribute to problems, especially raw foods.
- Investigate probiotic capsules and other organic supplements that can help you.
- Everyone's different, so you may have to experiment to find what works for you.
- Try working with a good nutritionist to figure out solutions.

Sleep

Did you know that the amount of sleep of our ancient ancestors followed seasonal light patterns? The human body produces chemicals regulating sleep according to input from light sources.

The internal mechanisms that regulate sleep and wakefulness make up a remarkable system. However, a variety of internal and external factors can dramatically upset the balance of this sleep/wake system. The amount of sleep we obtain generally decreases and becomes more fragmented as we age.

The modern human isn't that much different on a cellular level from our primitive forbears. Just over one hundred years ago, we learned to schedule sleep according to factory shifts made possible by artificial light. Today, we expect our sleep to conform to our needs and demands, regardless of our bodies' natural cycles.

Due to the invention of the electric light, we are now exposed to much more light at night. This new pattern of light exposure affects our sleep patterns.

Exposure to light in the late evening (TV, computers, e-readers, lamps, blue and green LEDs) tends to delay the sleep phase of our internal clock and contributes to some of us opting to go to bed later. Exposure to light in the middle of the night may make it difficult to get back to sleep.

Sleep Problems

Most people we talk with seem to have their own assumptions about how much sleep they need. Aging seniors complain about not getting enough of it, as well as not being able to get high quality, deep, refreshing sleep.

If noise is a problem for you, you probably have good hearing—and at least that's good. Sleep interruptions could be helped by a good pair of ear plugs.

A wide range of medical conditions have an impact on sleep. Such conditions as chronic pain from arthritis, leg cramps, frequent need to urinate, and gastroesophageal reflux disease are common causes of interrupted sleep. Moreover, the medications we end up taking to treat our various conditions also play into digestive and sleep problems. Excessive gas leads to farting and burping and can awaken you (or your partner). Not drinking enough water leads to dehydration and headaches which disturb sleep.

Prescription drugs have varying effects on sleep. Some of the things that can decrease the amount of REM and slow-wave sleep are alpha and beta blockers for high blood pressure, congestive heart failure, glaucoma, migraines, and antidepressants. See your doctor about these problems so you can find other choices.

And I haven't even mentioned annoying signals from our brains. Anxiety, depression, fears, and loss of loved ones affect many seniors. Some report nightmares. Even the most psychologically healthy seniors must face the realities of mortality and disabilities that come with age. Sleep is right up there as a number one major complaint in seniorhood.

Sleep Medications

One natural solution that we've adopted is melatonin supplements. I take five mg and Rob takes

10. We are more likely to get some good REM sleep when we take it. Ask your doctor and go online to research the side effects of prescription sleep medications, as many of them can be addictive and affect memory.

Alcohol

Alcohol is commonly used as a sleep aid. However, although alcohol can help a person fall asleep more quickly, the quality of sleep is compromised. Drinkers beware and be informed. Irregular sleep isn't the only bad result with regular drinking. It raises the risk for dementia and Alzheimer's. Yes, I know, small doses of red wine are recommended for health and longevity. It's just that few drinkers are truly moderate to the degree they say, from my observations.

Alcohol also tends to worsen the symptoms of sleep apnea, which further disrupts sleep. It can lead to more serious problems like dementia (not to mention that it disrupts others sleeping in the room).

Insomnia

It turns out that a sleepless night may cost you more than a morning of grogginess. Scientists at UC Berkeley's Sleep and Neuroimaging Lab have discovered evidence that missing deep non-REM sleep may leave the brain more vulnerable to memory loss associated with Alzheimer's disease.

(Alzheimer's disease, one of the most pervasive and debilitating forms of dementia, has been diagnosed in more than 40 million adults to date.)[2]

In the long term, chronic sleep deprivation may lead to a host of other health problems, including obesity, diabetes, cardiovascular disease, and even early mortality.

Don't ignore your need for quality sleep as you age.

ROB SAYS

Essential Sleep: Your body has a built-in diurnal rhythm, which is regulated by the daytime hormone cortisol, which governs your stress responses, and the nighttime hormone melatonin, which is produced by the pineal gland. People lose their natural melatonin beyond the age of twenty—particularly people above the age of 40 or 50 who produce little melatonin. There are huge variations depending on how much stress is in one's life. The more high-strung a person is, the more stress, and the more difficult it will be to fall asleep and sleep through the night.

On top of that biological component, there is the question of good or bad habits. Some people have no problem disciplining themselves to go to sleep between 10:00 and 11:00 p.m. Others are so used to their late-night activities (reading, watching TV, being online, playing video games, and writing novels) that they finally drop into bed at 1:00 or 2:00 a.m. Seniors need at least seven to eight hours of good sleep. Going to bed at 1:00 or 2:00 a.m. makes it difficult to get enough shut-eye.

What are the effects of going to bed late every night? A lot of hormones are reset during the deepest phase of sleep, triggered by melatonin. Even our telomeres, those caps on chromosomes in every cell, get shortened with stress and too little sleep, and shortened telomeres mean a shortened lifespan.

Here is one solution: because seniors undoubtedly have a decreasing supply of melatonin, the first step is to take 5 to 10 mg a half-hour prior to bedtime.

There are other natural supplements such as GABA (500 mg strength) available at health food stores. GABA combined with melatonin should help in more than 80 to 90 percent of insomnia cases. Of course, always check with your doctor first. Melatonin and GABA are safe. Prescription sleeping pills have multiple side effects for seniors, including memory problems.

Sleep Deficit

Anyone who has ever racked up a nasty sleep deficit knows that it ruins your capacity to recall information. There's a good reason for this. During deep sleep—also known as slow-wave sleep, when the brain is experiencing non-rapid eye movement—memory "traces" become reactivated, which triggers communication between the hippocampus and the cortex.

The communication between these regions of the brain helps maintain the neuroplasticity that is required to "cement" long-term memories in the cortex, which can be retrieved hours or years later.

Trying to induce those slow waves in the brain with a sleeping pill is tricky—and getting it wrong could possibly exacerbate memory problems. Experts advise that the easiest way to overcome sleep issues is to exercise regularly.

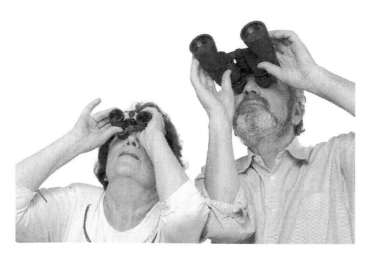

6   Eye-Opening Research

Our environment is much worse than it was in the mid twentieth century, and it's not getting any better. Our air, water, food, and ecosystem are overloaded with toxins and pollutants. This overworks cells, especially those of the immune system and liver.

Liver disease is a rapidly growing problem for seniors. More than one in three adults has liver disease, and if one drinks or has hepatitis, the risk increases dramatically. When 200 people were tested for pollutants in their blood or urine, 111 chemical substances were found in at least 60 percent of those tested.[1]

The buildup of these toxins over the years destroys our immune system and renders the liver dysfunctional. As if these attacks from our environment weren't enough, the food processing industry is slowly, methodically killing us.

My earliest recollection of a processed food was when General Foods created Maxwell House instant coffee, a product that was supplied to soldiers and ultimately introduced to the public in 1945.

From that time until the 70s, I had never heard the term obesity, while today some 35.7 percent of adults are considered obese with 68.8 percent labeled overweight.[2] Not to sound like one of those old farts that says, "In my day…" but, in my day, we walked to and from school, had physical education classes, plus before- and after-school sports. We brought our own lunches and ate whole foods, except for a few processed treats like chips or M&Ms—and there were almost no fast food joints.

We might not be able to influence a change in our environment during the few years we seniors have left. Some of us don't have the energy we had in the 1960s to fight the establishment. And yes, time is running out. We can advocate for cleaner air and fewer chemical ingredients in our food, but realistically, that might not be enough. It doesn't appear that we can depend on our political leaders to listen to science, medical research, or any one of us aging citizens (unless we're a lobbyist with tons of money funded by big corporations).

So, what can we do to fight the good fight, extend our health spans, and not give in to the war on aging? We can change the things we can change. We can take care of our personal hygiene, exercise programs, nutritional needs, and refuse to eat the processed crap they sell out of food factories. It's up to us, the foot soldiers in the war on aging.

PATSI SAYS

Medical research estimates that physical exercise and healthy habits can prevent 50 to 70 percent of chronic conditions of aging and reduce the effects of injuries and illnesses common to seniors.[3]

For example, when a group of seniors participated in a moderate amount of cardio activity each week, one study showed new growth of brain cells in MRI imaging. Other studies show a correlation between exercise and reduced risk of dementia and Alzheimer's.[4]

Rob and I don't want to beat you over the head with tons of research data, so we put some interesting studies in the appendixes. If you're a reader who wants to know the sources, you'll find them listed there along with books we recommend for learning more.

Safety First

When seniors start an exercise program, however, we really need to proceed wisely. That's not always easy to do; we either go too easy or too hard, and often don't use common sense when it comes to exercise and our aging bodies. When you think about it, how would we know what's prudent anyway? We've never been this old before! Most of us aren't trained in exercise physiology or healthcare. I advise taking a beginner's mind and where possible start with a physical trainer. Start right, start smart: get a professional to set up an exercise program with you.

Working out as a senior is a bit like learning to drive a car all over again. Don't drive too fast, follow the rules of the road (posture and form), and STOP *before* you feel the pain of a wreck. In other words, our advice to fellow seniors is this: don't spin out and crash because you think you're smarter, fitter, and younger than you really are. (That's something I tend to do more often than I admit!)

No matter your age, pay attention to your attitude and self-talk. Don't convince yourself you're too old, too tired, or too clumsy to learn to exercise.

The body dictates to the mind how it feels and it can change by the hour. Upon rising, we can feel stiffness due to how we've slept or just because it takes longer to get the blood circulating to joints. A few hours later, we might feel more invigorated. In the afternoon, we can contract a "second wind," or in other cases, we're just too tired and exhausted, and end up taking an afternoon snooze. Later that day, we eat dinner, read a book, or spend an evening on the couch watching Netflix—which can easily turn into another nap!

Remember, it's all in our minds. We tell ourselves stories about the energy we feel (or don't feel). So much of what we experience is created within our own brains. The stories we tell ourselves about how tired we are can stop us from engaging in life-extending exercise. Alternatively, what we tell our selves can propel us toward a lifestyle of strength and self-confidence. All we need to do to change our mindset is to change our self-talk.

I don't believe many seniors would opt to keep their sedentary habits if they knew what some of the medical research is showing. To me, it's worth a change in diet and exercise if we can live longer and stronger.

Do regular exercise and nutritious food help us live longer? There's only one answer: YES!

So, it's now or never. Our clocks are ticking like crazy. In some diabolical conspiracy, the hands of time seem to increase with speed and determination with each new year. Birthdays and anniversaries come at us at a breathtaking pace, as most of us continue to use our lousy excuses, instead of treating our bodies and minds to a better, healthier life.

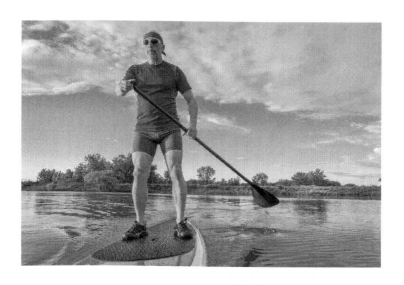

7 All One Body

Let's face it: *no one's getting out of this alive.*
Make the most of your body and mind during this
third phase many people call the golden years. Stop
yakking about how old you're getting and think
about how much better you will feel, think, act,
behave, and yes, even look, once you make a firm
commitment to a healthier lifestyle.

You're never too frail or too old to exercise. If
you're old, exercise can help you avoid bone loss

(osteoporosis) and muscle loss (sarcopenia). Exercise also improves your balance and dramatically lowers your risk of falling.

Combined with proper diet, exercise helps you shed excess pounds. And you don't have to hit the gym and sweat buckets; it really can be done gradually.

Exercising will in fact provide you with more energy. Exercise improves your circulation and causes your body to produce endorphins, which make you feel better. For me, once I get to that magical point of two hours of vigorous exercise per day, my body continues to burn calories long into the day and evening. Even at 70 or 80, your body can become a fat-burning machine of extraordinary proportions.

Yes, it can be hard, especially at first. But you know it doesn't have to be punishing for it to be effective. All you need to do is start moving by walking, swimming, or even dancing.

Do you know what's even harder than exercise? Getting sick from the lack of it. My personal experience with finding the time for vigorous exercise is typical. At the age of 39 (half my current age), I had a young family, a suburban home, and a sedentary career as an advertising agency copywriter. There was little time in any day, including weekends, to carve out two hours, or even a half-hour, for exercise.

Of course, always check with your health practitioner before starting any exercise program. But note that some medical practitioners underestimate the importance of exercise and fitness for older patients. While one should always consult a physician, seek out a doctor who is knowledgeable in sports, aging, and longevity.

Assuming you are still with us, you may be saying, "I already exercise because I walk my dog or stroll through the park every day with my spouse or friend." And some may be saying, "I'm not overweight, why do I need to exercise?"

Sorry to break it to you, but leisurely walks with your partner or your dog, unless you run free with your dog, do not qualify as "vigorous exercise." Plus, the reason seniors need to exercise is far more important than simply losing weight. It's about staying alive and functional.

At this point, after only a few years of dedicated diet and fitness, Patsi has achieved *Senior Fitness 4 Life* status. As a Super Senior (over 70 years), she and others like her know what that requires: commitment, time, and certainly dedication. The results are measurable but not only by the bathroom scale and the tape measure. The really important results show up internally. These are the benchmarks of our health platform. So, what does that all mean?

Here's one list from our website
www.seniorfitness4life.com

Senior Fitness 4 Life Benchmarks

- ✓ Increased bone density
- ✓ Lowered heart rate
- ✓ Lowered blood pressure
- ✓ Reduced cholesterol levels
- ✓ Better balance
- ✓ Greater endurance
- ✓ Stronger heart muscle
- ✓ Lower body fat percentage
- ✓ Added muscle mass
- ✓ Improved and deeper sleep
- ✓ Reduced risk of Alzheimer's, dementia, Parkinson's
- ✓ Increased self-confidence
- ✓ Increased mental and physical energy

Yes, those are lofty goals and some seniors may be skeptical that they can achieve any of them. But the truth is—and history shows many examples—we can change our life at any age. Most seniors can achieve *Senior Fitness 4 Life* status, and with some dedication and consistency, they can achieve it in less than two years.

PATSI SAYS

Whoa! Did Rob say, "the magical point of two hours of vigorous exercise per day?" That may be fine for him and other athletic seniors, but don't be discouraged. I started exercising later in life, with small efforts, and minimum time in the gym. It has built up over the last few years. Now, I (almost) enjoy working out, and I get more results in less time.

I'm often in and out of the gym in a half-hour. That includes a 10-minute warm up on a cardio machine, and 20 minutes of weightlifting on machines and barbells. So, no, I don't spend two hours on vigorous exercise a day like Rob does. (But I will easily spend two hours playing tennis, and because it's so much fun, the time flies!)

I think most senior women, and many men as well, must decide what's "vigorous" for them. What it usually means to doctors is activities that raise the heart rate to 60 percent or more of maximum. That is sweat level. For us, the key is to regularly engage in sports or an exercise that brings pleasure, fun, AND works muscles, heart, and mind. That can be gardening, dancing, or playing frisbee with the grandkids.

For Rob and me, it's tennis. That usually means playing three sets in two hours. If power walking with a friend or Fido gets your heart rate up, then that's vigorous exercise, as long as you do it for at least 20 minutes. That's how heart monitors and step trackers help. Trackers show if we're really getting enough exercise or just fooling ourselves.

In general, women are more likely than men to eat healthfully and be nonsmokers, but are less likely than men to be sufficiently active. In most of the research studies, older adults tend to be nonsmokers and eat relatively healthfully, but are more likely to have a high body-fat percentage and to be less active.[1]

* **

For those seniors who don't want to join a gym for whatever reason, we use the term "gym" as a metaphor for any place you choose to exercise, be it a park, a pool, a yoga class, a bicycle lane, a Pilates studio, a tennis or pickleball court, or a running track.

It's not what or where you exercise but how much and how often that counts. In the early throes of your commitment to exercise, it's more important to find activities that offer movement and fun and are playful in nature.

That's why we love tennis. You run, stop, go, hit the ball (hopefully) and then repeat that process again and again. It is a sport; it is play. You can keep score, and if it's important to you, you can win. There are many other activities that offer play value masquerading as exercise, and all these take your mind off exercise you may perceive as boring or repetitive.

Whatever activity or sport you choose, one does not need to be a natural-born athlete to enjoy tennis, pickleball, golf, water aerobics, volleyball, or an hour in the gym. The important thing is to get out there and do it! No matter your age or condition, you will find others who want to enjoy themselves too. Most medical doctors will tell you that exercise is the one prescription for health and longevity that doesn't cost much and has few side effects.

The Benefits of Aerobic Exercise

Aerobic exercise—also called cardio or cardiovascular workouts—includes jogging, swimming, cycling, walking, dancing, and anything that gets your heart rate up. Known to reduce anxiety and depression, this type of exercise boosts mood, in part by increasing blood flow to the brain. Exercise affects the hypothalamic-pituitary-adrenal (HPA) axis and, thus, reduces stress. This involves several regions of the brain, including the limbic system, which controls motivation and mood, the amygdala, which generates emotional responses to stress, and the hippocampus, which plays an important part in memory formation as well as in mood and motivation.

There are many benefits to well-being from exercise, including self-confidence and social interaction. Other benefits from your exercise plan are:

- Improved sleep
- Increased interest in sex
- Better endurance
- Stress relief
- Improvement in mood
- Increased energy and stamina
- Reduced tiredness and increased mental alertness
- Weight reduction
- Reduced cholesterol and improved cardiovascular fitness
- Increased focus and concentration

In any case, whether you indulge in aerobic exercise, resistance training (weights), or stretching and flexibility (yoga, Pilates, Tai Chi), all exercise has been found to alleviate symptoms such as low self-esteem and social withdrawal.

The Benefits of Strength Training

Strength training—also called resistance training or weight lifting—focuses on firming and building muscle. For seniors and anyone over the age of 50, it is the best way to stop the loss of muscle that gradually erodes our bodies each year. We mentioned sarcopenia before. Although it's a naturally occurring process of aging, you have a lot of control over the rate at which you lose strength and muscle over your lifetime.

It's not just something we should attend to for aesthetic reasons. Sure, muscle definition makes a body more attractive. More importantly, maintaining strength can prevent falls, slow down loss of bone density, and ensure we seniors can enjoy life to the fullest.

Here's the key to successfully maintaining muscle strength. It doesn't matter if you go to a gym and lift barbells, dumbbells, use a machine, or do sit-ups or pushups at home. The key is to lift weights that are heavy enough so you can do ten repetitions and repeat each series for three to four sets. If it's too easy, the weight isn't enough. If it's too difficult, use lighter weights. This simple formula for repeatedly lifting a weight will firm up muscles over time if you are consistently doing it two to three times a week. Even if you aren't building muscle, you are at least maintaining it.

Furthermore, the stress on muscles during resistance training affects the overall strength of surrounding tendons, ligaments, joints, and bones.

Strength training diminishes bone loss. Some studies show it may even stimulate bone growth. Bone density happens on the cellular level, which, even if we fully understood the biochemistry, we would have a hard time explaining to you. Just know that any time you're flexing and using muscles, as in a strength training routine, extra-heavy housework, and some sports, you are slowing bone loss that occurs in the aging process—providing you engage muscles sufficiently and beyond what's required for normal tasks.

When your muscles are in good shape, you can stop yourself from falling and prevent bone fractures. Weight training will help your strength and balance so that when you do trip you'll recover your equilibrium and stop falling all the way. Here's the formula:

Good muscle tone + balance + flexibility = fewer falls and fractures

---

Your Life Is in Your Legs

Legs are the wheels of the human body. They are the primary vehicles for mobility, for balance, for stability, and a driving force behind a healthy, active way of life. Functional legs are critical in maintaining a vibrant lifestyle as well as preventing injury and disability, particularly among seniors. The best options for keeping your legs in good shape are for you to get up, get out of the house, and start moving.

Here are just a few positive benefits for leg muscle training:

- Improved balance
- More calories burned (your whole engine runs faster)
- Lower back pain relief
- Increased range of motion/flexibility
- Reduced risk of falling

Without strong, healthy, and flexible legs you will wither away and eventually die. You will end up being dependent on caregivers or family members instead of having the freedom of movement you enjoy today. Walking, running, or bouncing on a mini-trampoline will add vitality to your entire body. Yes, it's true; your life is in your legs.

Your Second Heart Is in Your Stomach

On the surface, this statement sounds almost as absurd as *your life is in your legs*. But trust me, having a fit midsection, or body core, is crucial for increased longevity. As we age, the waistline seems to leave on a journey all its own. We have trouble sitting up as well as buttoning up. Over time our youthful V-shape turns into an O-shape, or worse, an OO-shape.

A weak core frequently leads to a weak back, and a weak back can cause us days, weeks, or a lifetime of pain and discomfort. If you suffer from back pain, it is likely that your stomach muscles need strengthening. The good news is that it's not too late to turn it around. In fact, it's never too late to get fit. We are never too old or too infirm to start rebuilding our core.

According to the Mayo Clinic, people who store fat in the stomach area are at high risk of stroke, heart disease, high cholesterol, diabetes, insulin resistance, snoring, difficulty sleeping, certain types of cancers, and other diseases.[2] There are two types of stomach fat. Fat which can be felt under the belt is called subcutaneous fat or superficial fat. Fat that lies deep inside the stomach, which can interfere with the function of the liver and other organs, is called visceral fat.

ROB SAYS

Years ago, I played AAU basketball as a guard. My best friend, Alan H., our point guard, was a tremendous athlete with gifted vision and uncommon court sense. Unfortunately, he was never in top condition and tired badly at the end of every game. He loved his burgers, Cokes, and fries, and over time he collected more than his share of belly fat. His strong legs allowed him the ability to compete, while his ample belly fat impeded his peak performance.

After a few years of losing to teams that weren't in our class, Alan and I had a chat about his conditioning. He very much wanted to improve his endurance to be a better teammate and, more importantly, become a vital part of our offense in the fourth quarter. At the time, he was in amazing cardio condition, having ultra-strong legs and, therefore, no amount of gym, cardio, or strength work was going to improve his belly fat condition.

The only salvation for his belly fat was a diet change. He gave up breads, pastas, fried foods, and sugars in the form of soft drinks and replaced them with a sensible diet of fruits, vegetables, nuts, legumes, and water...lots of water.

The next year, a very svelte Alan H. led the league in scoring and assists and the North Hollywood LDS went on to play in the National AAU Championships.

* * *

Strong core = strong back. If you are among the many seniors with back pain, be sure to strengthen it with an appropriate level of core exercises. Start with those you can do without pain, and work up gradually as your comfort level expands.

Of course, sit-ups alone won't be effective unless you also reduce calorie intake and avoid processed foods and hidden sugar. Think about exercise and diet as a two-pronged strategy to fight aging and ward off chronic conditions.

Routines for Strength

The miracle of weight training is that it slows muscle tissue and bone loss associated with aging. In fact, it is even possible to regain muscle that has been lost from years of inactivity. Cardiovascular training and stretching have their place in a balanced fitness plan, but it is progressive resistance exercise that builds muscle, allowing us to stay young, active, and independent for as long as possible. *Nothing else comes close to being as effective.*

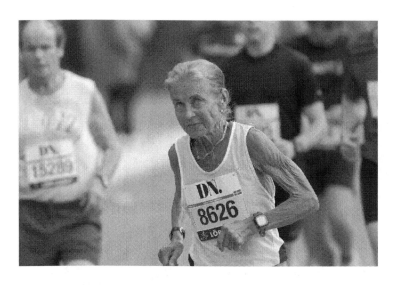

8   Why We Don't Exercise: Caveman
Brains

The answer to why we don't like exercise may be found by looking at our ancestors, the cavemen and women who bequeathed our genes to us. Yes, we are blessed with a genetic motherboard that's at least 10,000 years old, and without any upgrades to the operating system. If we were computers we would have blown a circuit board and crashed long ago.

But here we are, still functioning and adapting, still surviving after all these years on a caveman's brain. Cavemen (and women) were strong and lived by their wits. It was kill or be killed. We were either running after prey or running away from it.

In between, we rested, recuperated, and restored our energy reserves inside our cells. To do that, the body developed a hibernating-like conservation system. The human body is designed to expend energy and then conserve it selfishly.

A Genetic Bias

Cavemen never had to motivate themselves into action. Hunger motivated them. Dangerous prey motivated them. They never had to exercise self-control over eating. They ate as much as possible to hold them over during winters or famines so they would be ready for the next hunt.

Biologically, we still depend on danger or high stress to get us into gear. Otherwise, we love to relax and conserve energy. The brain tells us we need to rest until the famine is over and the tiger has passed. We have a built-in genetic bias against wasting energy. Why should we do sit-ups or squats? Wait for the tiger. Until then, relax.

Override the Caveman Brain

The senior caveman of today needs to override this genetic bias for relaxation and not let it get in the way. Smart seniors know they can do a number of things to avoid the vegetative urges to watch TV and eat junk food.

Endorphins

Use exercise to generate energy, drive, and get into action. Yes, I know it may seem paradoxical, like telling a depressive to "just do it." (Don't feel like exercising? Then exercise.) But exercise does produce magical chemicals like endorphins, your body's own opium. Once you get going, you can experience some intense pleasure. Just get started and let it happen.

Play

Combine exercise with playful activities you naturally enjoy. Make sure your exercise program generates pleasure. This means sports, games, and a variety of physical movements like yoga, dance, kayaking, or something you've never done before.

Consistency

Not to repeat ourselves and state the obvious, but before you can get hooked on exercise, you must start doing it and keep at it. Somewhere down the line you will learn to love it. Give it a chance to take hold. Persist, insist, and resist giving up.

Like our ancestors, we prefer to rest until we absolutely must move to get out of danger. Rest and recovery led to a survival advantage for early tribal humans. We learned to conserve calories and store them as fat when food supplies were limited.

Our ancestors didn't need to develop discipline, willpower, or self-control to motivate them to move. There wasn't an excess of readily available food like there is today.

Once we understand that we have the same caveman brain built to survive in more primitive times, we can use that information to our advantage. We can shift our thinking from "Why don't I love exercising?" and start asking "How can I overcome the urge to vegetate?"

Simply coming to the full realization of these facts can be liberating. When you don't blame yourself for being inadequate, you have more energy available to figure out how you will motivate yourself, despite going against a human nature that's outdated.

The enemy isn't your laziness. You may be trapped by a genetic predisposition to being sedentary. Sedentary habits aren't bad. We need to relax, restore, and repair. We need to sit to read books, be entertained by TV or computers, and to socialize and eat good meals with friends.

Yet too much time being sedentary will counteract all your good efforts at the gym and on the sports fields. It makes no sense to go out and play three hours of tennis and then sit the rest of the day. Yet that's what our brains will tell us we need to do.

How will you overcome those urges? It's eye-opening to track how much time you spend sitting per day as opposed to walking and moving around. Activity trackers make it easy to get accurate readouts on your steps and other physical measurements. Here's how one of our friends overcame her resistance to exercise by doing what she loves best.

Sally's Story: Reluctantly Fit

Is it possible to join the senior fitness movement without becoming a fanatic? Can you still have an active social life? This was a big issue for my friend Sally.

Sally M., a 69-year-old female, weight 160 lbs. and height 5'7", with a BMI of 25.1

- Had not exercised in years except for yoga and stretching classes

- Had never used any type of exercise equipment (e.g., treadmill, bike)

- Very high cholesterol and blood pressure (currently on meds)

- At high risk for obesity, osteoporosis, arthritis, and diabetes

- Bone density measures borderline for osteoporosis

- Needs to lose weight, improve muscle tone, balance, and stability

- Needs to reduce belly fat and lower her BMI

Sally is a fun and energetic woman who loves friends and social gatherings. She always hated gyms and exercising. However, she was propelled into thinking about fitness when she unexpectedly divorced and wanted to start dating. She scheduled an appointment with a weight-loss doctor and had a physical exam prior to cosmetic surgery for a face-lift.

Both doctors told her the same thing: if she didn't change her lifestyle, no matter how young her face looked or how much weight she lost, she was at high risk for heart disease and diabetes. Furthermore, she'd lost bone density and any fall would probably result in fractures.

Working with a wellness coach, she identified two activities that she enjoyed: walks with friends and dancing. She joined a local weight-loss group where she could socialize with new friends. After two months, she agreed to reconsider an exercise program at a gym.

Eventually, she found a group of friends to go to the gym with, started working with a trainer, and then augmented her gym routine with two days a week of walking one mile at a normal pace. She began tango lessons and went dancing with a weekly senior singles group.

Sally discovered that a Mediterranean diet, which allowed her to "cheat" one day per week, worked well for her. During the first year, Sally increased her walks to two miles, twice a week. She still didn't like the gym and eventually dropped out. She replaced it with a senior Zumba class, which gave her great cardio exercise and helped with weight loss.

After one full year, due to her dedication, Sally's BMI dropped to 21.1, and she lowered her weight from 160 to 135. Her risk for obesity and diabetes dropped into the safe zones. Sally acquired much better balance through dancing, and is careful about not falling.

Her cosmetic surgery was a success. She recently met someone online, then had several in-person dates and decided to play the field for a while. She says she now has confidence in herself, both inside and out, and feels for the first time like she's in charge of her health.

Sally changed her life.

Give Exercise a Chance First

Sally wanted a quick fix for aging, and opted for cosmetic surgery. But she soon discovered that she wanted more than just to look good. She wanted to feel good, too. She discovered a way to exercise that she enjoyed (dancing) which fit in with her social life.

Even with cosmetic surgery, you'll need an exercise program which you should start well before you have surgery.

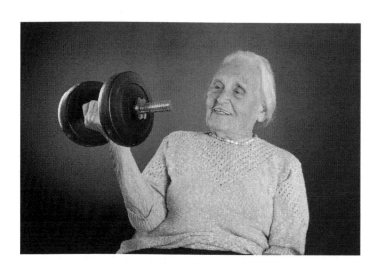

9 Why We Don't Exercise: How to Use Goals

PATSI SAYS

Given all we know about the benefits of exercise, don't you find it curious that most people don't like to exercise?

My husband and I are in the meager 2.7 percent of people who make exercise a regular part of daily living. That percentage is even lower for people in their 70s, which we both are.

Every survey and health study we researched report dismally low numbers of people who regularly engage in exercise.

According to the U.S. Health and Human Services, 74 percent of adults over eighteen don't exercise regularly. Forty percent don't get any leisure time exercise at all.

Another resource reports that less than five percent of adults participate in 30 minutes of physical activity each day.[xv]

More than 80 percent of adults do not meet the minimum guidelines for both aerobic and muscle-strengthening activities.[xvi]

Only 25 percent of people aged 65 to 74 say they engage in regular physical activity.[xvii]

We don't find many seniors who disagree they should exercise more or who don't know how important it is for health. The problem isn't knowledge. We know we need to exercise; we're not stupid, at least not generally. If you have lasted 50 to 65 years or more you probably aren't an imbecile, weak, lazy, self-destructive, or suicidal.

Yet, to *not* engage in regular exercise *is* suicide, albeit a long, slow, debilitating, and painful way to go.

And since most of us are not suicidal, then why don't we like to exercise?

Two Obstacles to Exercise: Injuries and Not Seeing Results

I've seen a lot of women get on the exercise bandwagon and fall off early because they started something too intense, got injured, or they worked their tails off without seeing physical results.

Either way, you're not likely to sustain a healthy exercising habit if you get hurt or work hard for nothing. However, consider this: even if it seems like you're not getting results, you are.

Internally, your blood, heart, liver, and lungs all benefit, and of course your brain improves too. Many of the benefits of exercise aren't seen superficially, but science assures us that key changes start happening on the cellular level.

Lack of results is a major reason people stop working out. Here's an example from my own experiences: for years, I went to the gym and did the same routine, always the same four or five machines, three sets of 12-15 repetitions, some arms, legs, butt, and abs. (Oh, and 45 minutes of cardio so that I could still eat junk food and not gain weight.)

I always did the machines I liked, that were easy for me. I put them at 10 or 12 lbs. so I wouldn't have to strain or sweat. I rarely increased the weight settings. After a few months, I'd get bored and stop going. Then when I went back, I'd start over again at the same machines with the same weights.

Occasionally, I'd complain to a personal trainer who'd show me some other machines or some free weights and work the sweat out of me. I'd go home panting and sore, and convinced I'd found the solution. Then I'd be back in the gym, three to four times a week, doing the same old things all over again.

I never worked with free weights (only the guys did that) or increased weights, or tried the things that felt like a strain, so with the same efforts, I got the same mediocre results. Duh!

At least I never stopped doing the cardio machines. Those kept my legs and heart and respiration in good shape. (And I still ate junk food.)

I mention this because I've talked with other women who do or have done the same thing. Today I see plenty of women in the gym who hit only the treadmill or elliptical or bike machines. Some do only the jazzercise or Zumba classes, while others prefer yoga. But increasingly, I see a few women performing bicep curls, shoulder exercises, and core work. I believe that's a new trend because women are getting smarter about the need for a more comprehensive approach to physical well-being.

Strength Training for Women

Still, we have a lot to learn. Most women don't understand the importance of strength training for aging well. They still think it's only for the guys. I know plenty of women who believe yoga is sufficient for staying healthy. One yoga friend just had surgery for multiple fractures to her wrist, incurred as she fell and broke the fall with her hand. While yoga is great for keeping a body young and supple, it doesn't always have the same weight-bearing benefits for bone density that strength training does.

I love yoga, and I love doing cardio (despite how hard it is to get started sometimes). I didn't like working out with free weights at first, but now, after a year, I'm learning more about it and seeing results. I love it.

I felt a hard bulge at the back of my arm the other day. It was my triceps. I'm working body parts I never have in the past, like my biceps and shoulders. And being able to feel muscle definition where flab used to be is a great motivator!

Because that's what we do as humans; we are pleasure-seeking animals at our core. And we are also one of the few mammals who can and will delay gratification if we see a more important goal in the future. Not everyone is practiced and skilled at this, but we can become so.

What separates the talkers from the doers is action. I don't know many people who *don't* struggle with starting to exercise. And those who start it often drop out because it's hard to sustain any habit, especially an exercise or dietary habit.

There are always good reasons to put it off. I mean *really good reasons* that are impossible to deny. Life happens.

KISS: Let's Keep It Simple, Seniors

You don't have to take on every form of exercise in the gym and become a fitness expert or gym nut. When I mentioned before that even the most disciplined and intelligent among us struggle with health habits, I am not kidding.

Take out some insurance by using a few smart tools. Let's call it "Goal Insurance," although it really is another type of life insurance, one that will extend the quality of your life.

To use Goal Insurance requires you to write down your exercise goals, but in a way that is different from the usual SMART goal technique. Remember the SMART Goals System? Goals should be written out to be:

S = Specific
M = Measurable
A = Achievable
R = Realistic
T = Time bound

For the *Keep It Simple, Senior Goal Insurance Plan*, I want you to first write down a stretch goal for your exercise plan. A stretch goal is something you dream of being able to achieve, but don't really think or know how you could do it.

Stretch-plus-SMART Goal Plan

Here's an example of my friend Jan's stretch goal and how we made it into a Stretch-plus-SMART goal plan. At first, Jan came up with this:

Acquire an almost daily cardio exercise routine.

First off, you can see how this misses the requirement of SMART goals. What cardio exercise will she do? What is "almost daily"? How do you measure "acquire"? How will she know when she's accomplished this? It's not bound by time. I asked her to rewrite it as a true stretch goal.

Jan argued back that participation in any daily cardio routine would be a huge stretch for her. Even one week would be truly amazing, or even a series of three days in a row. I agreed, and after more discussion and some arm twisting, she rewrote the stretch goal followed by an action plan based on the SMART criteria.

STRETCH Goal: I want to complete a half-marathon walk in a year.

97

SMART Goal: Within six months, I will have completed 30-minute walks six days out of every week. Within nine months, I will walk 60 minutes six days a week. At the end of 12 months, I'll walk a half marathon of 13 miles.

Specific: To start, the first week I will walk 10-20 minutes at a slow pace for three out of seven days. Each successive week, I will add one or two minutes, walk faster, and add one day a week until I am up to six days a week and I can do a half mile in under 30 minutes.

Measurable: I will use my Fitbit tracker to measure days, time, steps, miles, and minutes.

Achievable: Based on previous experiences, I know I can achieve this. I will use a walking buddy to help ensure motivation.

Realistic: Because of getting support through my friends, and having had a recent medical checkup, I know I can realistically do this. I believe I can do more, but want to accomplish this first before raising my level.

Time-Bound: Yes, I'm giving myself a year by breaking it up to weekly, monthly, and six-to-nine-month time frames to build a consistent record.

You can use this same goal plan for any type of exercise goal. If you want to lose weight, you will probably want several goal insurance plans, one for food, one for exercise, and one for stress, emotional factors, enjoyment, and play— whatever is an obstacle for you.

Just remember to keep it simple, seniors. You don't want to complicate things and make fitness a burden. Remember, a bird doesn't build a nest with one twig.

ROB SAYS

Like most people, I used to think I didn't have time to exercise. Today, I *make* time for exercise. As a result, I have more energy and less stress and find that I generate more creative juice to follow my passions: writing novels, painting, sculpting, public speaking, business mentorships, and university lecturing around the world.

I co-founded Razer at age 56. I founded MindFX Science at age 60. I didn't start writing until age 65 and I've now published seven novels (this is my eighth book). I began guest lecturing on marketing and technology at age 75.

Because of my exercise regimen, I find that for every hour I exercise, I have an additional three hours a day of creative energy to pursue my interests.

Not bad for a *Super Senior*! Am I lucky? Yes, AND I put in the work to earn it. Will I live forever?

Certainly not. The doctors say they don't know how I ever survived my heart attack in 2004. And they are baffled by what I do physically and how I maintain my daily regimen.

There are always going to be health challenges: strained muscles, joint pain, and degeneration of various parts. The trick is to adjust and work with what you've got. There's always a way to incorporate more movement into your life.

It's hard to prove that I've extended my longevity because of my health habits, but then again, I really don't want to find out what happens if I stop.

How to Confront Excuses and Do It Anyway

Here's how I motivate myself. Whenever I find I don't want to go to the gym or whatever, I review my reasons for setting these goals, examine the obstacle, and remind myself how/why I will do it anyway.

Exercise or Sport	Why I want to do it	What will stop me	How I will do it anyway
Tennis	Competition, social aspects, winning, fun.	Rain and assorted aches and pains. A	When it rains, I'll spend more time at the

		third heart attack.	gym. It's really an addiction.
Gym workouts	Feel good, feel strong, and feel confident. Releases pleasure hormones.	Tend to over-train, injury, need for rest. Often tired and hungry before I get to the gym.	The same reason they climb Mount Everest... because it's there.
Cycling	Strengthens legs and improves heart and lungs.	Cold, rain, and muddy roads. Traffic.	Being outdoors in nature (what's a little rain?).

Achieving goals can be a powerful motivator in a senior's life. Some of us love striving for goals, such as learning a language, playing a new instrument, or living to 100. We need to achieve and our motivation is piqued by accomplishing challenging tasks quickly and effectively.

When it comes to our core intrinsic motivations, age is no barrier. Age is merely a limitation we impose on ourselves. As basketball coach Pat Riley said, "There are only two options regarding commitment. You're either IN or you're OUT. There is no such thing as life in between."

Are You IN or OUT?

It's easy enough to commit to the idea of staying healthy and exercising, and it's easy to say we believe it's good for us, will prolong our lives, will improve our looks and how we feel. Who doesn't want that?

But true commitment that lasts is all about finding the core reasons you want to make changes. What really matters to you? Do you want to look better for your spouse? Feel better? Live longer, maybe be around longer for your grandkids or your great-grandkids? Dance better? Have better sex? Increased confidence?

Find out what truly matters to you and make that commitment to do what it takes.

But here's the thing: it's easy to commit and say you'll do it... tomorrow. The urge of the moment—for feeling good right now—will override the desire for feeling good at a later point in life. You will reach for the TV remote or the French fries and beer to get instant pleasure. You will put off exercise; that's a given.

Why not borrow a few tips from recovering alcoholics who've rebuilt their lives by changing habits? People who stop drinking are told to commit to only one day at a time. Don't drink today. Sometimes they think in terms of one hour at a time. It's hard when you think about forever; you only have to do it now. Tomorrow's another day. You can change your behavior only one step at a time anyway.

H-A-L-T

One of the most common moments when people chuck their good intentions happens when they are hungry, angry, lonely, or tired... or bored. Instead of being hungry, angry, lonely, or tired, why not go for a walk? Recovering addicts use this H-A-L-T tool all the time.

While you can't avoid strong emotions, you can respond differently to them. Find something to do that takes you away from these feelings. Exercise just happens to be an excellent way to channel negative into positive energy.

Phone-a-Friend

Learning to HALT and change habits often requires some help from a friend. Recovering addicts use the power of social relationships or sponsors to help them. If they want to pick up a drink, they're told to pick up the phone. Call someone with experience in breaking bad habits. Use the power of other people to help get over the humps. You can do this to respond differently to unhealthy triggers for food or sloth.

Yes-You-Can

Don't let faulty assumptions trip you up. When you tell yourself "What's the use? I've never been able to do this in the past," you're ignoring the fact that you've never been here before. What I mean is that you've never been this experienced in life as you are now.

Or, as a Hallmark birthday card put it, "Hey, you've never been this old before, but think of it this way: you'll never be this young again!" So, gather what's left of your motivation, willpower, and strength and put them to use NOW. It's only going to get harder next year.

Let's Eliminate the Obstacles

While thinking about your motivations, you will want to consider possible obstacles and plan ways to overcome them. The most common barriers seem to be:

Time

For many of us, being too busy is the big obstacle. How can we find time each week to exercise? You might consider combining strength training with another activity or with a social visit. Instead of going out to lunch, lift weights with a buddy or family member. The half-hour or so that you spend watching reality TV is a perfect time to sneak in a whole workout.

Maybe the best way to overcome time impediments is to treat exercise as a job and assign your workouts as such. Think, *I have a two-hour-per-day job, five days a week, and I must be prompt or I will fire myself.*

Fatigue

It's a proven fact that strength training gives you more energy; it also makes other daily activities easier. This fact can help you override your fear about being too tired or not having enough time. If you really feel tired, tell yourself you will commit to starting the activity for five to 10 minutes and then re-evaluate your energy levels. You may surprise yourself.

Age or Fitness

If you think you're too old or out of shape to lift weights, rest assured, people have successfully started strength training in their 70s, 80s, and even 90s, and you can too! And if you believe you won't live that long, Social Security historically has recorded 6.5 million people in the U.S. who have lived to the ripe old age of 112. You just might find yourself one day celebrating a 100th birthday. You want to be fit enough to be able to blow out those candles and enjoy those added years!

If you are not active, you need to start slowly and follow basic safety rules. There is no such thing as being too old, too feeble, or out of shape to benefit from strength training.

Health Concerns

If you have a health problem, talk to a health practitioner before you start any exercise program, of course. Chances are, your condition will not stop you from strength training, although you may need to make some adjustments. In fact, you may be among those who gain the most from this form of exercise. We remind you that you should never exercise if you have a health condition that is unstable or serious, or if you have new symptoms, or your doctor recommends against it. If a general practitioner advises against weight training, get a second opinion. Some doctors are more informed than others about the benefits of exercise and diet on longevity.

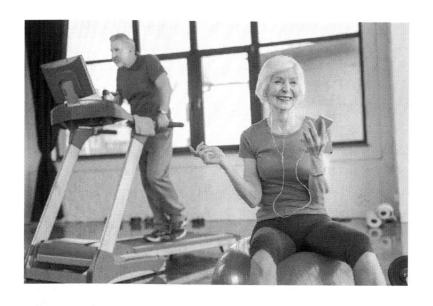

10   Suiting Up: Rob

An often forgotten yet important part of the starting steps in the Senior War on Aging is to invest in proper gear and equipment. First step: proper shoes.

Your oh-so-comfy casual sneakers are not the best footwear for more demanding use in sports, and certainly not for spending time in the gym, on the treadmill, or even out walking. If you're running, get a running shoe; if you're playing tennis, get a shoe made expressly for tennis; and so on. Active sports require better support for feet, ankles, and Achilles than any cool-looking pair of Skechers.

The same theory applies to apparel. You should plan to sweat, so get loose-fitting, lightweight, quick-drying clothing with wicking qualities. You don't want material that will chafe your skin or shoes that will cause blisters. Regular cotton t-shirts will quickly get wet, sticky, and heavy if you're getting your heart rate up and sweating (as you should if you want to get both heart and brain benefits). Instead, try the "dry-fit" materials engineered specifically for sports activities.

Proper hand protection such as workout gloves, golf gloves, and any other accessory for your specific sport will save on blisters and calluses. There's a reason they invent these accessories, besides just looking good. Buy some wrist sweatbands so your hands remain dry and headbands so sweat doesn't get in your eyes. And of course, helmets and headgear for bicycling and motor sports are vital. The same goes for eyewear protection for cyclists and swimmers. Use a sports cap or visor and sunglasses to protect your eyes from strain and harmful sun rays.

You don't have to spend a lot of money to get proper gear, so treat yourself and protect your hands, feet, and skin. If you're out in the sun, don't forget a good sun block with a minimum SPF 30 level. Look for "water resistant" sun block since most activities induce sweat.

Feet, Don't Fail Me Now

As we age, our feet become more sensitive to pain, calluses, and injuries, which is why we recommend paying a little extra for good athletic footwear. Each foot contains 26 bones, 33 joints, and more than 120 muscles, ligaments, tendons, and nerves. These all work together to support the weight of your body, act as shock absorbers, keep you balanced, and push you forward with each stride. With the additional stress to your feet, don't skimp on better quality, superior fit, premium athletic footwear.

Every time your foot strikes the ground during tennis, running, or any impact sport, a vertical force equal to approximately two and a half times your body weight is transmitted through your physique. This is called *vertical ground reaction force,* and if you think back to your physics days in school, Newton's Third Law tells us that for every action there is an equal and opposite reaction. When the foot strikes the ground, you drive a force down through the foot. In reaction to this force, the ground impacts a force back up through the foot and leg. This force is called the *ground reaction force.* So, at 194 pounds, every time I run on the tennis court my feet are dealing with 485 lbs. of kinetic energy through my athletic shoes and up through my ankles, knees, hips, and lower back.

My sports watch calculates that I take a minimum of 4,000 steps per day on the tennis court and I play every day. That's a cumulative 1,940,000 pounds of impact per day! Now tell me if you still want to run in those stylish Skechers you bought at the mall.

Sock It to Me

Before you try on a pair of high-performance athletic shoes, first give serious consideration to proper socks. Yes, even socks can make a huge difference to your feet. What you want in an athletic sock is moisture-wicking material, arch and toe cushioning, and good materials that "breathe."

Make sure to wear sports socks when trying on athletic shoes for fit, as they can make a difference in the size or model of shoe you choose. There are also many over-the-calf compression socks available for seniors with calf muscle and vein problems.

For tennis, I prefer seamless toe socks for maximum comfort. Most cheaply-made socks have a rather pronounced ridge in the toe seam that can cause calluses, blisters, chafing, and bunching.

You should also consider compression briefs, shirts, tank tops, socks, sleeves and joint braces for ankles, elbows, knees, and lower back, all of which can help support your body—injured or healthy. These form-fitting garments are often made from a spandex-type material. The main benefits of compression sportswear are that it keeps your muscles warm to prevent muscle strain and fatigue, and it wicks sweat away from the body, thus preventing chafing and rashes.

At least when you dress the part, you'll look good and feel motivated, if nothing else! Having the right shoes, shirts, shorts, and compression wear will get you in the mood for exercise even before you're out the door.

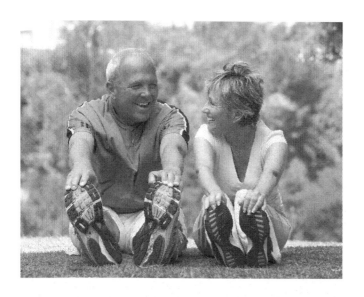

11   How to Exercise: Rob

Everything you do to move and enjoy yourself while exercising will create healthy habits that are good for your body, brain, and all the way down to your mitochondria! Even when you don't think all this work is working for you, it is; you just can't see it inside your cells.

Yet there is one type of exercise that stands out above the others in terms of creating younger-looking bodies and actual younger-acting cells: strength training.

Strength training with weights, also known as resistance training, is exercise that involves lifting, pushing, and pulling against a force, usually a dumbbell, barbell, or other piece of equipment.

Starter Techniques: Machines or Free Weights?

Machine workouts are simpler, safer, and easier to learn to use. Most machines have pictures affixed showing what to do and which muscles are involved. This makes them easy to use on your own, and you can create your own circuit. You can also figure out what to do simply by watching the person ahead of you. And you can always ask a gym employee or fellow member about the proper use of any apparatus.

Machines are designed to isolate muscle groups efficiently. Since the body is stable on machines, one can target large muscle groups effectively. Make sure you position yourself properly and adjust at a low weight to start.

Machine workouts allow people to progressively train with heavier weights without assistance. This isn't the case when using free weights (dumbbells and barbells). With machines, you can easily add extra weight without risk of injury, so they're perfect for working out alone, without a partner or spotter. (Note: proper technique is still paramount before you start adding weight, so train smart.)

Machines are useful for older people who may be weak from lack of activity or who may be in rehabilitation after injury or surgery. Machines will get your strength up quickly and safely.

One of the worst things I see in the gym is men and women using machines incorrectly. In an attempt to add a little more weight, they fail to use the full range of motion the exercise was designed for. Instead of moving all the way up and all the way down, they use momentum or other muscles to jerk the weight partially up and down, with short bursts of energy, often using less than half the range of motion the specific exercise requires. Not only does this minimize the benefits of the full motion, but it often places strain on the back.

Consider using lighter weights with a greater number of repetitions, better form, and full range of motion. Remember that we're older now and supposed to be wiser! There is little satisfaction in trying to keep up with others in the gym. Leave that to the testosterone-pumping young studs. Start light, go slowly, and aim for full range of motion. Lift smart!

Machines are designed to do each movement with control and very slowly. Slow movements toward contraction, a pause at that point, and slow movements toward extension, and then a pause at the resting point. You should set the machine at a weight that can allow you to accomplish ten repetitions using a full range of motion with slow and calculated movements. The muscle you're using should feel some stress or burn for the last two or three repetitions.

You must learn to use your breath properly during each exercise as well. Breathe out as you lift or push a weight and breathe in as you relax. Don't hold your breath during strength exercises. Be in control: don't jerk up and then allow the weight to fall. These are all good reasons we advise starting an exercise program with a personal trainer.

Why Dumbbells Aren't for Dummies

Free weights consist of dumbbells, bars with weighted plates, and weights attached to cable pulley machines. With free weights, you can use a fuller range of motion—you have complete freedom to move around rather than being locked into a specific range of motion or pattern like on the machines. This allows your body to do what it is naturally built to do: move freely. With free weight movements you engage smaller muscles, ligaments, and tendons surrounding the joints, to stabilize the movement.

This extra work is how lifting free weights keeps joints healthy and strong when done properly. You are strengthening all the components of a joint as well as the muscles. This is important as we grow older, lose some of our natural balance, and become prone to tripping or falling. Strong joints mean we can catch ourselves and avoid a full fall.

In my opinion, free weights provide more bang for your buck. If you have limited time to train and want to get a lot accomplished with few exercises, then free weights are the way to go. But you may need to start with machines to build up some strength first.

You can also vary your routine with free weights. With machines, you are limited to what each machine is designed to do. One machine usually works only one set of muscles. With free weights, all you need is one dumbbell and you can do hundreds of different variations: pulling, pushing, circles--you name it. You can do compound exercises involving several body parts and muscle groups, as in dead lifts and lunges.

Also, when you've learned to train with free weights and use your own body weight, you can train anywhere. Machines and equipment aren't always available. When we go on vacation and travel by car, it is easy to bring a kettlebell, some elastic bands, and some light dumbbells to get in some quality training.

Free weights are also the way to go if you don't have access to a gym since they are much less expensive and take less space than machines. You can easily build a basic home gym for under $200.

Nevertheless, we highly recommend joining a gym and starting with machines or a mix of machines and free weights before advancing to a more intense resistant weight-training program.

One of the many advantages of hiring a personal trainer is to get a customized training program specifically suited for your age, body, and current condition. A trainer can guide you until you understand enough about your body to avoid injuries. Start with a good exercise program designed specifically for you, follow that for a while, and get ready to upgrade your workouts to super senior fitness standards.

Now, I am aware that many seniors do not want to join a gym. There are many reasons for this. Still, I want to encourage you to join one, especially to get started. Here's why.

Most gyms have simple exercise machines that help you get started correctly. I would seek out gyms with newer equipment. As the science of exercise advances, engineers are designing and improving machines to advance performance. Ergo, the newer the machine, the better it is for your fitness comfort, safety, and control.

Most gyms have personal trainers who can develop a custom-designed exercise program for your age, gender, physical condition, and level of fitness. The trainer will monitor your form and development, helping you achieve optimum performance level. Perhaps the best thing about a personal trainer is that you need not sign up for a long series of sessions. If you wish, the trainer can get you started for one to three sessions, and then you can decide to continue on your own—or, as I recommend, with a workout partner.

I encourage you to visit your local gyms before you sign up, more so for previewing equipment than for price. Most gyms will be competitively priced, particularly for new members. Look for gyms offering cardio equipment, free weights, and the latest in exercise machine technology. Some gyms have very new equipment and provide towels and liquid in spray bottles for members to clean the equipment after each use. Others are "muscle gyms" with a lot of testosterone and banging of free weights. I do not recommend that type of gym for any beginner—in fact, after many years of gym life, I don't like those gyms even for myself.

Look for a clean gym with an assortment of new or newer machines, a limited number of (relatively light) free weights, and populated with people like you. Visit a gym during peak hours (early morning or late afternoon) to see how crowded it is and the type of members (gym rats and muscle-man posers or people like you).

Ask to meet with a personal trainer and request a couple of beginner sessions. Then, if all is to your liking, sign a gym membership for one month (unless you are 100 percent committed to this program and their yearly or senior discount is favorable). In many cases, daily memberships are available, which allow you to decide if this is the place for you before you enter into a longer contract.

Assuming you have a workout partner, have invested in proper footwear and workout apparel, have found an acceptable gym, and signed up with a personal trainer, what can you expect?

Early Days at the Gym

First, ask your trainer how many days a week you should schedule your sessions (we recommend starting with a minimum of two days per week). You can also ask your trainer what he recommends, given your health, preexisting conditions and fitness level. This is important so that your trainer can establish a routine suited to your age, current level of fitness, and which body parts to focus on (or protect) during each session.

Your trainer should start you off with a five- to ten-minute warm-up on a bike or treadmill, at a very slow pace. Then he will demonstrate proper form for arm, chest, shoulder, and leg machines or free weights, using lower weight settings to gauge your strength and the amount of time it takes for you to recover from each exercise.

Ask your trainer to document your routine in writing (most of them automatically keep a log of your routine) so you can have a record of machines, settings, weight levels, and number of repetitions for each exercise. Over time you will increase the weight and number of repetitions, including lessening the time between sets of exercises.

Logs are an excellent way of tracking your progress and for recalling which machines and what weight settings were used when you last worked out. Along with strength and endurance, there are unseen benefits you may want to track on your own.

The three most crucial benchmarks for seniors are bone density, muscle mass, and body fat. I encourage you to obtain a baseline test before you begin your exercise program. Note that most personal trainers can test you for body fat and BMI (body mass index).

As I mentioned before, expect some muscle soreness after your initial workout. Trust me, there are some muscles you have not used since the Great Flood and they will be tested. Do not allow a little after workout stiffness and soreness to slow or stop you from your next scheduled workout session. The second time around you will have little or no soreness because you've begun to strengthened the muscles. And the longer you maintain your exercise program, the less soreness and stiffness you will experience following each session.

These baby steps should eventually lead to greater mental and physical energy that will help motivate you toward taking the next big steps.

Form and Technique

When using machines or free weights, exhale while you take three seconds to lift or push a weight into place, hold the position for one second, and inhale while you take another three seconds to return to your starting position. Don't let the weight drop; return it slowly under control.

A personal trainer or workout buddy can monitor your form and help you maintain an even pace. While it is nice to have someone there to chat with, what you should be concentrating on is an even pace and proper form. Save the social hour for after your workout.

Again, breathe out as you lift or push a weight and breathe in as you relax. Don't hold your breath during strength exercises. This could affect your blood pressure, especially if you have heart disease. It's surprising how many people don't realize they hold their breath.

Focus on your form. Use smooth, steady movements to bring weights into position. Avoid jerking or thrusting movements, especially with your back. Try not to use body momentum and swinging the weights. Always lift well within your limits. There is no reason to push your muscles to exhaustion— leave that to the body builders on Venice Beach or in Gold's Gym.

A word about weight training and heart disease: so many of the men and women I know who have suffered heart attacks and strokes have a fear of lifting weights or even raising their heart rate through cardio exercises. The American Heart Association says, "Just as we once learned that people with heart disease benefited from aerobic exercise, we are now learning that guided weight training also has significant benefits."[1]

How to Build Strength

To build strength, gradually increase the amount of weight you use. Start out with a weight you can lift only 10 times. (That means you start to have difficulty maintaining good form by the tenth time.) Use that weight each time you work at that exercise until you can lift it easily 10 to 15 times. It may take you a few days or a few weeks. For some, it may take longer before you can comfortably raise the weight without losing proper form.

When you can do two sets of 10 to 15 repetitions easily, add a little more weight so that, again, you can lift it only 10 times before your form starts to fail. Repeat until you reach your goal. Usually, the goal is three or four sets of 10 to 15 repetitions for each exercise.

Limit recovery time between sets. In the beginning, you may want to time your recovery period and limit it to 30 or 60 seconds. You shouldn't rush through your routine, yet the benefit of limiting rest time between sets is enormous.

This is the way muscle strength is built over time. Forcing the muscle to contract and extend to its fullest ability damages muscle cells. For regaining or building strength and muscle, damage is a good thing. That damage is what provokes the repair process that adds additional strength and builds more muscle tissue. Muscle soreness is the result of stressing the cells so that they need to repair themselves.

This is why you should not work the same muscle groups two days in a row. Give your muscles time to generate the chemical reactions necessary for cellular repair.

Don't just guess how many repetitions, number of sets and how much weight you complete during each workout. Track what you're doing so that at your next workout you have a record and a starting point from which to record your progress.

Alternate days you work each of the major muscle groups. The muscle groups forming the upper body are the abdominals, pectorals, deltoids, trapeziuses, latissimus dorsi, erector spinae, biceps, and triceps. The major groups of the lower body are the quadriceps, hamstrings, abdominals, and glutei (the butt).

Muscle soreness and some fatigue are normal after muscle-building exercises, at least at first. After a few weeks, you should not be all that sore after your workout. If you give your muscles time to recover, you can train every day by alternating which areas you work.

For example, an advanced routine might look like this:

Day 1: Legs and Abs
Day 2: Chest
Day 3: Back and Abs

Day 4: Rest

Day 5: Shoulder and Abs

Day 6: Arms

Day 7: Rest day or stretching

Admittedly this five-day split is for more advanced seniors. It is designed to get the three toughest days done when you're fresh, and to separate chest exercises from arms to allow your joints to optimally heal. This is the split I use.

Tips for Sustaining Exercise Habits

Do you know what really works, not just when starting to exercise but also for keeping it up? Find a friend who will commit with you!

Get a buddy as your workout partner. Having a fitness companion is often the key to:

- Getting your mind off activities you won't always love
- Maintaining an even pace to your exercise
- Motivating each other to work harder
- Bringing you both back on a regular basis

For seniors who have been sedentary for many years, having a friend or workout partner can make the difference between maintaining a regimen and quitting prematurely. Most of us are social creatures who need the camaraderie of other humans. Do not underestimate the importance of the social side of fitness.

It's also safer to have someone to monitor your form, track your sets and repetitions, provide constructive feedback, and for general safety reasons. The most common cause of injuries (at any age) is bad form, which can be hard to determine if you work alone. For me, I want someone to spot me when I'm lifting heavy weights. Same goes for sports. With friends, we can motivate each other.

"I would never join a club that would have me as a member" Groucho Marx

---

Early Days on the Field or Courts

Assuming you opt for a more playful or non-gym approach, what can you expect? Much of this depends on your play activity.

Tennis requires more gear and equipment, but it offers a mix of cardio endurance and stop-and-go aerobics (interval training), and requires some leg and upper body strength to wield a racquet and drive the ball with power.

Cycling also requires an investment in gear and equipment, and is excellent for endurance and leg strength. It is fun, scenic, and, like tennis, offers great exposure to vitamin D. If the great outdoors is inaccessible due to weather, most gyms offer stationary bikes and/or spinning classes.

Both Pilates and yoga can be a wonderful total body workout mixed with meditation and mental focus, plus excellent joint-relief stretching. For most seniors, yoga offers limited endurance training, nor does it build muscle mass, but it's a great way to build joint strength, flexibility, and balance—keys to preventing fractures and falls. It's also an excellent place to meet people.

Golf can be a great fitness primer, but only if you walk the course and heft your own golf bag. Like tennis and yoga, it can be social and you can likely find a regular partner. Personally, if golf were my play activity of choice, I would arrive at the course first thing in the morning with a few balls and tees in my pockets and begin alone, carrying only a five-iron—and run the course while playing. (But then, that's just me!)

Other excellent forms of play are:

- Pilates
- Zumba
- Pickleball
- Line, ballroom, jazz, and tap dancing
- Hiking
- Jogging
- Power walking

- Martial arts (Tai Chi and Qi Gong)
- Swimming
- Water aerobics
- Volleyball
- Ping-pong
- Exercise videos (can be rented from the library or available online)

While these are all great for getting started, many lack full-body workouts, which is why I recommend adding resistance training to your sport or activity of passion. Additionally, you can enhance the energy and play factors of these activities by adding music. Here are other ways to make exercise more like play than work:

- Listen to music while lifting weights, running, or on cardio machines
- Get competitive while playing tennis (keep score and win)
- Take photographs on a nature hike
- Meet new people at a yoga class, fitness center, or at the tennis court (convert them into workout buddies)
- Watch a favorite movie or TV show while on the treadmill, stationary bike, or elliptical trainer, or read or listen to books on tape

- Instead of chatting with a friend over coffee, chat while jogging, power walking, or strength training
- Listen to music while power walking the golf course
- Run with a dog—it can be as good for you as it is for the animal. If you don't own a dog, offer to take a neighbor's dog for a run or volunteer at a pet shelter
- Go for a run, power walk, or cycle when you're feeling stressed and see how much better you feel afterward
- Find an exercise buddy--someone whose company you really enjoy and try activities you've never tried before; you may find something new to love. At worst, you would have spent time with a good friend
- Use personal trackers like Fitbit, Garmin, Jawbone, or smartphone apps like My Fitness Builder

Personally, I recommend music as a cathartic and invigorating exercise tool. Upbeat, hard-driving rock (I prefer 80s rock) can become a great motivator while exercising—during both aerobic and resistance training. Music can help you power through tough exercises while relieving your mind of the tedium of repetitive routines.

Home gyms are a great way to get started or convenient for days you can't make it to a real gym. They don't have to be decked out with fancy equipment, either. Stretch bands are inexpensive and you can use household items for resistance training.

Set up your home gym in a room that allows you to escape interruptions, like a basement, garage, or simply any room with a door you can shut. It helps to have a full-length mirror to monitor your form. If you don't have dumbbells, fill large soda bottles with water and perform a variety of exercises that make you raise the weights above your head, out to your sides and in front of you.

Practice exercises that require you to move and maintain your balance, if you're able. For "young" seniors in their 50s, 60s, and even 70s, perform workouts that simulate the aerobics classes at a gym. Try hopping, quick dance steps, or a step aerobics workout. Do half-squats and lunges while holding dumbbells or resistance bands, bending down as low as your knees will comfortably allow.

Take time to stretch your muscles after each workout to help prevent later stiffness and soreness, and to improve your flexibility. Don't "bounce" while you stretch, to prevent injury. Move your muscles just past their point of natural resistance and hold them there for 15 to 30 seconds. Save this type of stretching for after workouts, since stretching before resistance training temporarily decreases your strength and you can get injured.

For our home gym, we have invested in a professional elliptical machine, stretch bands, pushup handles, and lightweight dumbbells. Patsi and I use the elliptical trainer nearly every morning before tennis to warm up. The other items are for the days when our gym is closed, such as Sundays and holidays.

One of the reasons I highly recommend a real gym, over or in addition to the home variety, is motivation. There is something magical that happens to my inspiration levels when I enter a gym having a multitude of free weights, cardio equipment, and exercise machines. I am highly motivated by other people who are building body, mind, and spirit. I am much less motivated working out by myself at home.

Cross-training and High-Intensity Interval Training (HIIT)

Cross-training is typically defined as an exercise regimen that uses several modes of training to develop a specific component of fitness. For example, if you want to improve your ability to hold a pose in yoga, you might want to build leg strength with weights or machines. Cross-training for tennis might include working on cardio fitness, and a good way to do that would be to include high-intensity interval training (HIIT).

HIIT is gaining recognition as a fast-track method to build overall fitness and lower risk of chronic diseases. New research shows that even six minutes a week of HIIT brings far superior health results than 30 minutes a day of cardio activity at a steady speed. On the play side think of racquet sports as great interval training alternatives to the gym.

For example, instead of walking for 30 minutes on a treadmill at a moderate pace, you mix in 30 to 60 seconds of sprinting all out, then rest or walk normally, then continue injecting 30-to-60 second intervals of high intensity. Altogether, your cardio session may only be 15 or 20 minutes, but the three or four high intensity intervals provide maximum stimulus to cellular metabolism. Here's what the research shows, as reported by Dr. Mercola's health website:

- High-intensity interval training (HIIT) can significantly improve your health and fitness in mere minutes per week
- Health benefits from HIIT are largely due to HIIT boosting the number of mitochondria in

your cells, responsible for production of energy in the form of adenosine triphosphate (ATP), and improving their function

- Aerobic fitness is determined by measuring the amount of oxygen your mitochondria can consume when you push yourself to the limit, a measurement called VO2 max; the lower your VO2 max, the higher your risk of chronic disease.[2]

By including some cross-training activities in your usual routine, you acquire multiple benefits:

Reduced risk of injury: By spreading the level of orthopedic stress over additional muscles and joints, seniors can exercise more frequently and for longer durations without repeatedly overloading the same vulnerable areas of the body (e.g., knees, hips, back, shoulders, elbows, and feet). People who are particularly prone to lower-leg problems from jogging, running, or playing tennis should consider incorporating low-impact activities into their regimens, such as elliptical training, treadmill, cycling, yoga, and swimming.

Enhanced weight loss: Seniors who want to lose weight and body fat should engage in an exercise program that enables them to safely burn a significant number of calories. Research has shown that this goal is best accomplished when individuals exercise for relatively long durations (more than 30 minutes) at a moderate level of intensity (60 percent to 85 percent of maximum heart rate). Overweight individuals can effectively achieve a reduction in body weight and fat stores by combining two or more physical activities in a cross-training regimen. They can, for example, exercise on an elliptical trainer for 20 to 30 minutes and then weight train for an additional 20 to 30 minutes.

We've both known individuals who have lost substantial weight (50 lbs. or more) walking long distances—seven to 10 miles, two or more days a week. It can work for anyone who dedicates the time and who may not be able to run or do more vigorous training. The challenge is once they lose weight is sustaining their exercise and diet regimen.

Improved total fitness: Cross-training activities develop muscular fitness as well as aerobic conditioning. While a cross-training senior's muscular gain will typically be less than if he or she participated only in strength training, the added benefits of improving strength and endurance can pay substantial dividends.

Improved exercise adherence: Many people drop out of exercise programs because they become bored or injured. Cross-training is a safe and relatively easy way to add variety to an exercise program. In the process, it can reduce the incidence of injury and eliminate the potential for boredom.

Personally speaking, I have used cross-training techniques for years to improve my tennis game. Cross-training helps improve my footwork, lateral movement, and on-court endurance. I notice its benefits most when I'm away traveling for over a week. Unfortunately, when I return to the courts, it appears I have lost the physical edge of a cross-trained body—and it can take a few days to rebuild. As I've lamented before, getting old is not for sissies.

I also know a lot of golfers who cross-train regularly. Cross-training helps their legs and balance, and adds distance to their shots. Golf is a mind game where self-confidence makes a big difference, and being fitter than your opponent provides increased confidence.

Years ago, Patsi and I lived in a golf and tennis community in La Quinta, California. One of the golfers there complained to me that golf courses should have only 12 holes since he was exhausted for the last 6 holes. He would stand on the thirteenth tee dog-tired and his game would break down badly from that point on. I suggested he cross-train and accompanied him to my gym, put him on a stationary bike for 20 minutes, and then showed him a simple resistance program designed primarily for his core and legs. Before he began to cross-train he was a 15-handicap golfer. Not bad. Two years later he held a nine handicap and never tired on the course. He even bragged that he could now play up to 36 holes a day without fatigue. That was in the year 2000 and he continues to cross-train for his golf game three days a week.

I cannot think of any sports or fun activities that can't be enhanced through cross-training techniques. Swimmers, runners, power walkers, yoga enthusiasts, tennis players, and cyclists all benefit from weight resistance and cardio training to improve performance.

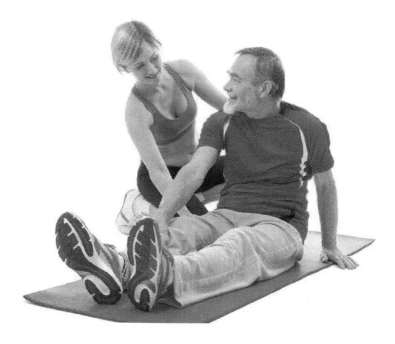

How to exercise: Get a trainer or a buddy

12 How to Exercise: Patsi

Cardio Warm Up

I recommend mixing cardio exercises into your weight training routine. Begin a warmup with five to 10 minutes on the treadmill, elliptical trainer, or stationary bike. It is not important which of these you select. Choose the one you most enjoy. If you like to read while doing cardio, pick one that makes it easy to read and has a ledge for your book, magazine, or e-reader. Some people like to watch TV and most people enjoy listening to music while they run, walk, step, or pedal.

What is important is to warm up your muscles, increase your resting heart rate, and prepare your body for the weight training routine that follows.

Over time you should increase both the resistance levels and the amount of time you spend on your favorite cardio machine.

You say this is boring? Spending 20, 30, or 40 minutes on one machine is tedious? I agree, which is why I often break my cardio training into three parts. Let's say I plan to dedicate 45 minutes to cardio. To make the routine more pleasant, I break it up and spend 15 minutes on the treadmill, 15 minutes on a spinning bike, and 15 minutes on the elliptical trainer. I use up-tempo music through my smartphone to help energize me and power through those tedious minutes. (I imagine you can tell that cardio is not one of my favorite exercise endeavors.) I also take my Kindle and read to make the time pass quickly.

The high-intensity interval training Rob talked about is a great way to avoid boredom during cardio exercise. You mix in short periods of fast pace with your regular pace. It makes the time go by faster, and with HIIT, you get increased health benefits after only six minutes of intense intervals.

I used to downplay the benefits of walking compared to jogging, but not anymore. Not only is walking better for knees and back, but the health benefits are comparable without wearing out any body parts.

I'm not downplaying the benefits of cardio training; however, know that your body at rest burns approximately 50 to 70 calories per hour, and that you will typically burn 250-300 calories in a 45-minute cardio workout. This seems to be a great deal of time and sweat to invest to burn an incremental 190 calories, which can be completely blown by consuming half a bagel.

For those of you who are looking to lose weight by burning more calories during your time in the gym, I recommend reversing your cardio and weight training routines. Weight training burns more calories because it is more stressful to your muscles than cardio. And, as you build more muscle tissue, your body fat decreases.

Weight training can burn calories for up to 39 hours following your workout. A cardio-first routine as a warm up is fine, but studies show that your body does not burn cardio calories until after the first 20 minutes. (Unless, of course, you are doing high intensity intervals.) If you lift weights for 30 minutes first, your body will burn calories as soon as you begin your cardio routine.

Weight Training Alternatives

This section may appeal more to women, but lately I've seen more than a couple of very fit, good-looking senior men in dance, yoga, and Pilates studios. They may be trendsetters, so secure in their masculinity that they're not afraid to try out new moves. (At least I don't think they are there to pick up senior chicks, but then again...)

Balance Ball: Above all, the most important part of your body to work out and strengthen is your core.

By strengthening your core musculature (all the way around your torso) you strengthen your back and abdominals, have better posture, AND LOOK BETTER!

I recommend buying a balance ball and using it for sit-ups, back, and core exercises. I've found that sitting or lying over a balance ball is the most comfortable way to do sit-ups. It's easier on your back and you get a full range of motion for your abdominal muscles.

Part of the reason that core exercises are so important is that when you work your core, you end up using all your other muscles, especially legs, hips, and back. This is essential to prevent falls and accidents.

Yoga Is for Every Body

Savvy women have been doing yoga forever, and the popularity of yoga classes keeps growing. For both men and women, yoga and Pilates are usually offered in group classes with professional instructors to guide you, aiming to improve your flexibility, balance, breathing, and strength as well.

Yoga is relaxing and good for relieving stress because it uses deep breathing with soothing music. The instructors gently guide you to achieve correct posture for the poses. You just show up with comfortable clothes and socks and follow their lead.

Please note, however, yoga is not typically a cardiovascular exercise, and you won't get the health benefits of raising your heart rate. If yoga is the only thing you do, consider adding another activity or sport, as, by itself, it may be insufficient. Unless, of course, you work at an advanced level and get your heart rate up.

Pilates Is a Unique Exercise System

If you're not familiar with the Pilates exercise system, try a class and find out how effective it is at improving body movements, stability, strength, balance, and overall well-being. When practiced with consistency, Pilates improves flexibility, builds strength, and develops control and endurance in the entire body. It emphasizes alignment, breathing, flexibility, developing a strong core, and improving coordination and balance.

Pilates is different from anything else you've tried. It is a safe system of mind-body movement using either a floor mat or a variety of equipment, such as the Reformer bed. It evolved from the principles of Joseph Pilates, a German innovator who taught dancers in New York. People swear by it, claiming it can dramatically transform the way their body looks, feels, and performs.

Pilates builds strength without excess bulk, creating a sleek, toned body with slender thighs and a flat abdomen. It is particularly effective at building core strength (abdominals, waist, and back).

My favorite Pilates classes are those using the Reformer beds. These are wooden torture-like-looking devices with cables for hands and feet. The base slides back and forth using spring-loaded tension cables of various resistances.

Professionally-trained instructors usually give classes, many of whom are retired ballet dancers. There's a reason trained dancers are attracted to Pilates. It provides both strength training and

144

stretching for muscles, but just as importantly, it engages many of the small supportive muscles surrounding joints and major muscles.

Dance: A Fun Way to Get Fit

Just because your doctor tells you to get in 30 minutes a day of heart-pumping exercise doesn't mean you must suffer in a gym or sports field. Dance presents a fun way to pass an hour and get the fitness benefits which prolong a healthy life.

Dance studios are everywhere and it's easy to join classes in everything from pumped-up hip-hop and Zumba to salsa and jazzercise. My favorite is tap dancing. You'd be amazed at how easy it is to learn, and you don't have to be super fit or graceful to start.

Check out the possibilities online or on YouTube.

Water Aerobics: A Fun Way to Get Wet

Water aerobics builds cardio, strength and resistance, all while being super easy on the joints and in a cool and relaxing atmosphere. It's also a great place to meet other energetic seniors. Believe it or not the resistance in the pool can range from four to 42 times greater than air, ensuring the body's muscles get a rigid workout. And with outdoor pools you derive the health benefits of vitamin D.

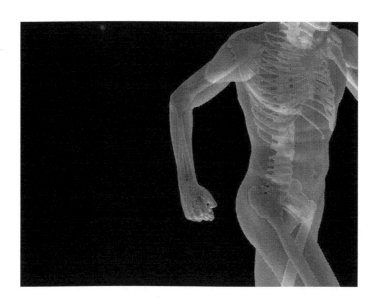

13   How Much Is Enough?

ROB SAYS

Scientists recommend 30 minutes of vigorous exercise per day, and to be honest, that just doesn't seem like enough. For me, I feel I require more than that...up to two hours per day.

What did I just say??? You're thinking, "*He's obviously referring to some world-class athlete and not us old folks. Exercise vigorously two hours per day? Who has the time and energy for that?*"

The point here is that I have been playing and exercising my entire adult life without prolonged breaks. No one expects you to start off that way knowing that your body requires time to adapt to the stress of rebuilding muscle and bone. Nearly anyone can commit to 30 minutes a day and if desired, build from that base.

In fact, fully- or semi-retired seniors may be the best demographic for this because most have the time to focus on fitness daily. So, I'm not bragging about my high level of exercise— what I'm saying is that other seniors 77 years of age can reach higher levels of fitness if they desire.

So many seniors believe that they are getting enough exercise by walking, wading in the pool, playing with their grandkids, their pets, or working in their gardens. I hate to be the one to break this to you, but those leisure forms of exercise don't count for much. To those of you who believe that you are getting health-redeeming exercise from leisurely strolls, I say it's a good start, but if you want longevity and health, add 30 minutes of heart-pumping and go for the sweat.

For an example of genuine life-extending exercise, my 73-year-old wife and I begin our day with 20 to 40 minutes on the elliptical trainer machine, located in our home gym, and then two hours of fun yet competitive tennis, five to six days a week, followed by an hour of weight training five days a week.

Admittedly, we did not start off at that level nor do we think you should. We built our strength and endurance over time. We now have a base of fitness where we can participate two to three hours a day without giving it a second thought.

Yes, there are still days when we struggle to force ourselves onto the bike or into the gym. Some days we just don't want to face a half-hour of morning cardio (the bed feels so warm and comfy), then two hours of tennis (my knees still ache from yesterday), and then to our local gym for weight training and stretching. Everyone has their own built-in reasons that they perceive as preferable to another hour of weights, machines, cardio, stretching, and sweating—and so do we. As do a few thousand of our friends.

Why do we do it, continually pushing our bodies beyond what appears to most people as compulsive—even neurotic? Quite simply, it's because it works for us, makes us feel and look younger, and strangely, we've grown to love it.

Here is the minimum senior fitness program recommended by the American College of Sports Medicine (ACSM) and the American Heart Association:

For muscular strength and endurance, a disease-free sedentary adult needs to use strength training at least twice per week, one exercise for each major muscle group to include legs, back, chest, shoulders, arms, and abdominal muscles. Lift weights approximately eight to fifteen times, gradually working up to 70% to 80% of your one repetition capacity; that is, a weight that you could lift only a single time. It is recommended that a very sedentary individual begin at an even lower level and gradually work up in intensity. The strength-training session need last only about 30 minutes.

For cardiovascular efficiency, it is recommended that one work up to at least 30 minutes of cardio exercise on most days. The exercise can be almost anything that will gradually raise heart rate and can include walking, bicycling, and many other activities, in or out of a health club setting. Sedentary adults can begin with as little as 40% of estimated maximum heart rate and work up to a range of 50% to 85%.

We now have a life expectancy that is more than double what it was 150 years ago simply because we have better hygiene, antibiotics, and medical procedures. Even so, we can't rely on science to fix everything. What's crucial here is to alter our health habits as soon as possible so that whatever comes our way we will have a fighting chance. We can all become soldiers in the Senior War on Aging.

Is Running Better Than Walking?

Apparently, there's no need to envy those fit fanatics who are still able to jog. As far as getting all the good health benefits for lowering heart disease risk, cholesterol, and blood pressure, walking may have an edge. This is according to a study whose participants were 18 to 80 years old.[1]

This is especially important to know because seniors may no longer have the knee and back strength for jogging. And, quite frankly, there are fewer excuses for not walking, right? Well, if you insist, but you'd have to be creative to think up good excuses for not taking a walk.

Pain Is Nature's Way of Telling Us to STOP

Be it resistance training, a long run, a bike ride, or a spinning class, if you feel pain, back off and STOP. I do not ascribe to the idiom *no pain, no gain*. That way of life might be okay for youthful competitive athletes, hell-bound on building mass by destroying muscle tissue first, but for our mature population pain represents significant danger. Best rule of thumb: avoid or modify any exercise that causes you pain or discomfort.

Don't mistake muscle burn for pain. In resistance training, the last few repetitions of any exercise should exhaust the muscle group you are using. That burn you feel is neither pain nor discomfort; it is muscle fatigue and that is the very best way to build strength and endurance. Be smart and learn to listen to your body.

How to Build or Regain Lost Strength

Big muscles come from lifting heavy weights (and usually assisted by taking drugs) and we do NOT want to start there. For seniors, the best way to begin the process of increasing or regaining lost strength is through more sensible body-weight resistance exercises.

Body-weight exercises are extremely convenient and effective. You don't need any equipment or gym, since you use your own body for resistance. For example, you can do push-ups in a variety of ways, depending on your starting strength. Do them against a wall, or on the floor when you are stronger. Women often push up from the knees or flank pushups until they can do a full-body floor pushup.

Because body-weight exercises are simple, and preventing injuries is easier, body-weight training is much more forgiving than other types of weight training. It is incredibly easy to modify to your ability level, whether you're a recovering couch potato or world-class senior athlete. Body-weight training helps develop better body control, balance, and proprioceptive awareness.

This form of exercise increases not only muscular strength but also muscular endurance, the ability to repeat a movement over and over. Although body-weight exercises can build a high degree of fitness, they do have limitations. Since a person uses his or her own weight to provide resistance, the weight being lifted is always the same, though the repetitions can always be increased.

Also, some seniors may not be strong enough to start with some of these exercises, especially if their body weight is excessive. For some women and seniors with little upper body strength, pushups and pull-ups may not be feasible. Here again is where a personal trainer can help develop alternative ways to develop upper-body strength.

Many seniors who begin to train have soft-tissue injuries. You should always speak to your doctor prior to beginning a new workout program.

Again, I highly recommend beginning your new workout regimen with a personal trainer. To start, they do an assessment, and you should disclose your physical limitations and injuries.

Can You Work Out While Injured?

Before deciding which exercises are safe, you and your trainer need to consider the technique used as well as your conditions, such as age, injury history, and current fitness level.

Be guided by your physical therapist, fitness instructor, and your doctor. If you have an injury or medical condition, talk with a sports medicine doctor, exercise physiologist, or physiotherapist first before embarking on any fitness endeavor.

As we age, changes in body shape, loss of muscle tone, and weight gain pose potential risk for injury. It is essential that all seniors discuss their exercise plans with an expert, as each body is different.

Be aware that increasing the speed, weight, or number of repetitions of any exercise can intensify the risk of re-injury.

I know I'm repeating this but it's important: avoid or modify any exercise that causes you pain or discomfort. Don't ignore your body's signals.

Consider cross-training with other fun sports and exercises to reduce the risk of over-training, particularly overusing injured or weakened body parts.

Make sure you have at least one recovery day, preferably two, between workout sessions every week. In the beginning it may take you more than the usual 24 hours to recover. It's not unusual for some seniors to need 48 or even 72 hours of recovery time. Conversely, don't lie to yourself and use minor soreness as an excuse to put off returning to the gym. Stick with your workouts— your life may depend on it.

This is one of the hardest things to discern: what is natural soreness due to good stress to a muscle versus what is a possible injury. When you start exercising, you may not be able to tell. Err on the side of safety at first. You will eventually learn what "good" soreness is that requires only time for recovery, and what is an actual problem that needs professional care. Learn to read your body and its signals. Remember that "real" injuries need rest—trying to "work through" the pain of injury can cause more damage to soft muscle tissue and delay healing.

Light workout cardio training is an excellent alternative for seniors suffering from existing injuries. Short five- to 10-minute sessions, two to three times a week, can help you maintain your fitness level while your injury heals.

PATSI SAYS

Here's a perfect example of trying to heal an injury without talking to a doctor. Or maybe I did, and he told me to stop playing tennis for a while. I had a torn muscle due to overuse while serving in tennis. My right shoulder hurt so bad I had cortisone shots which only masked the pain. Finally, I agreed to stop playing tennis altogether and let it heal on its own.

To my surprise, after four months of no tennis, I was totally unable to wield a racquet, swing and hit a ball, and serving was still impossible. I had lost mobility and was unable to raise my arm above my head. I went back to the doctor and complained, of course. I had thought I was doing the right thing, but my shoulder had "frozen," meaning scar tissue had formed, preventing normal use.

If I had been smarter, I would have spent those four months rehabilitating it with a physical therapist, who would have given me exercises to do to prevent buildup of scar tissue. As it was, I spent another four months breaking down the fibrous tissue in order to regain use of my right arm and shoulder. It never was the same, and six years later, I opted for surgery, with only moderate success. Live and learn.

ROB SAYS

Find Your Current Fitness Level

It's time to find your personal fitness level, which should help you understand the best approach to either starting or expanding your fitness goals. See if you can find the category closest to your age and current fitness standard:

- **Level 1**: Any age and currently having an existing injury: get an individualized program adjusted for your limitation or condition. A trainer can help you find what you can do, and explain how to train during healing.
- **Level 2**: Under 65 and currently inactive: begin a body-weight exercise program three days per week.

- **Level 3**: Over 65 and currently inactive: begin a body-weight exercise program two days per week.
- **Level 4**: Under 65 and having a low level of activity: begin an intermediate exercise program three days a week.
- **Level 5**: Over 65 and having a low level of activity: begin an intermediate exercise program two days a week.
- **Level 6**: Under 65 and exercising moderately more than one day per week: begin an intermediate exercise program three days a week and cross-train one day per week.
- **Level 7**: Over 65 and exercising moderately more than one day per week: begin an intermediate exercise program two days a week and cross-train one day per week.
- **Level 8**: Under 65 and exercising vigorously more than two days per week: begin an advanced exercise program (chapter 8) three days a week and cross-train two days per week.
- **Level 9**: Over 65 and exercising vigorously more than two days per week: begin an advanced exercise program two days a week and cross-train one day per week.

Note that the recommendations above are general in nature and do not take into consideration existing physical problems or deterioration, including lifelong tobacco or alcohol addictions. In other words, your mileage will vary. After you start exercising, you may find your recommended level too easy or too hard. Also note that you do not automatically become old on your 65th birthday—this is merely an equitable demarcation line, separating youthful seniors from super seniors.

These Fitness Levels are designed to help you to find a reasonable exercise routine for your age and existing activity situation. After testing the waters, you may find that you need to move up or down the ladder.

Lastly, the exercises attached to these Fitness Levels are all body-weight, cardio, resistance, and stretching in practice. If you prefer to substitute more playful activities, such as tennis, golf, volleyball, swimming, hiking, etc., just exchange the number of days recommended for your level. At the very least, consider one day of body-weight or weight-training exercises added to your playful activities.

For seniors, developing strength can be a double-edged sword. While it's certainly possible to rebuild your muscle mass and regain much of the lost strength from youth, there are also health risks involved. Besides the obvious muscle, tendon, and ligament pulls, there's the chance of heart problems and stroke. Therefore, before you begin any strength routine, please contact a sports medicine doctor, exercise physiologist, or physiotherapist.

What is sad to report is that large numbers of physicians are overweight and don't exercise regularly. Many physicians have little to no understanding of the benefits of exercise and do not realize that *exercise is medicine*. When embarking on a new exercise regimen you may want the second opinion from a sports medicine specialist.

On the positive side, strength/resistance training can also reduce the signs and symptoms of many diseases and chronic age-related conditions in the following ways:

- Osteoarthritis—Reduces pain and stiffness and increases strength and flexibility
- Diabetes—Improves glycemic control
- Osteoporosis—Builds bone density and reduces risk for fractures with falls
- Heart disease—Reduces cardiovascular risk by improving lipid profile and overall fitness
- Obesity—Increases metabolism to burn more calories and helps with long-term weight control

- Back pain—Strengthens back and abdominal muscles to reduce stress on the spine

Preference

People often enjoy strength training exercises and find them easier than long, tedious aerobic workouts and love the results.

Health and fitness benefits

Strength training can increase muscle mass and bone density. It makes you feel strong, energized, and confident, relieves stress and depression, and gives you a better night's sleep. It can also help prevent the onset of certain chronic diseases or ease their symptoms.

Improvement in appearance

Lifting weights firms the body, trims fat, and can boost metabolism by as much as 15 percent, helping to control your weight.

Social opportunities

Exercising with friends or family gives you a chance to visit and chat while you work out.

Thrill seekers

People who start strength training later in life often find that they are willing and able to try new, exciting activities, such as skiing, climbing, parasailing, windsurfing, or kayaking.

If more seniors participated in a regular program of weight training, they would see dramatic changes in their bodies and feel better both physically and mentally. Seniors who train with weights look younger than their age and are able to better handle tasks of daily living. They have more energy, fewer illnesses, and when they do get sick recuperate faster. They have lower risks of the common diseases associated with aging.

Even if you're on a regular aerobic program, we recommend you counterbalance it with moderate weight or resistance training.

The biggest challenge for seniors who want to get fit is to not overwork muscles and joints to the point of causing debilitating soreness and injury. You'd think that after living as long as some of us have, we'd know the limits of our bodies so well we wouldn't make this mistake.

Sure, we listen to our bodies when they go "OUCH!" But how many of us listen to the small signals leading up to *ouch*?

The Mind of the Warrior

Here's a sneak peek into the mind of a typical male warrior in the gym (raise your hands, ladies, if you know one of these). Listen to what this weekend warrior tells himself:

Hmmm, the last guy using this bench press had only 175 lbs. on the bar.

I'm much stronger than him; let's go for 200.

After all, when I was in college, I pressed 240 easily.

If I can do these 10 times, I'll keep going.

Wow, that felt good! I didn't even feel my bad shoulder, like the last time.

Here we go... 220... six, and seven, and eee-eight, NINE!

Okay, one more, inhale, exhale, grruntttt.... arghhh! (POP!!!)

Damn, my shoulder! What the ....!!!

The hard part about getting fit while being older is that it's easier to get injured and it takes much longer to heal. What we think we can do (based on memories, past experiences, and a past younger body) is misleading and dangerous. While a good self-image is important, unrealistic ambition is just plain stupid.

This is hard for many seniors to accept. We often need to lower our expectations to successfully improve fitness without injury. Many of us are reluctant to give up the competitive drives of youth in exchange for good common sense.

Wise seniors don't set themselves up for injuries to happen, or at least not often. They learn from their missteps. Listen to your body before it goes "OUCH!!!"

The Perils of Undertraining

The other side of the coin is the person who is cautious to the point that he or she undertrains. This is a waste of time in the gym. Being afraid to challenge yourself because of a prior injury or condition will not bring beneficial results. Your muscles need to be stressed to repair and grow. If you want to win the longevity lottery, you must at least buy a ticket.

The entrance ticket for senior fitness is doing something just about every day of the week that is challenging without being injurious. Like Goldilocks and her porridge, it must be "just right."

Goldilocks: What's Just Right for You?

Just as you're an expert who knows your own excuses and motivation, you are the only one to truly know your body and its amazing abilities and limitations. But, unfortunately, none of us are good at discerning what's enough and what's not enough when it comes to exercise.

You need to stress muscles enough to trigger the good chemical reactions within cells that will provoke the repair process and build strength.

But you don't want to overwork or damage muscle tissue. This happens when you go too far, either with too much weight, improper breathing or form, you run or walk too long or fast, stretch too quickly, and let your competitive nature get the best of you. It's easier to get injured as a senior because you're just not accustomed to your body's decreasing limitations. It's human nature to think we can do as much or more than we used to when younger.

But injuries can have devastating effects on seniors, leading to permanent disabilities, exacerbated conditions, and ruining possibilities for an active, healthy, and long life.

Even though we see many seniors not doing enough exercise to get life-extending health benefits, doing too much too fast without proper preparation is a huge obstacle to senior fitness.

Don't let injuries put you on the bench. Get savvy, know, and trust the signals from your body. Approach exercise with the mind of a beginner; after all, you've never been this old before. Make good use of trainers, physical therapists, coaches, and healthcare experts.

Proceed with caution, give exercise a chance to work, one step at a time, one push-up, one step at a time. Make this stage of your life the best one yet!

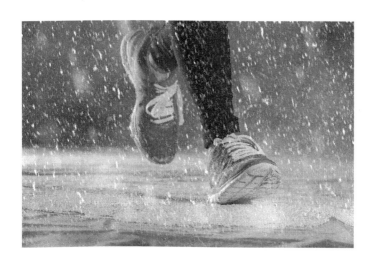

14   Cold Weather Training

ROB SAYS

My good friend Art Wannlund pointed out that most of this book centers around warm weather training. Since Patsi and I have spent the last twenty-plus years living in San Diego, Palm Desert, and now Ajijic, Mexico, it is understandable that our focus has been to enjoy exercising outside. We get up every morning, throw on a pair of shorts and get moving, almost always in warm weather. No need to consult the weatherman or even look outside; most of our days are sunny, with 70- to 80-degree temperatures year-round.

No matter what the temperature is, exercise and fresh air are crucial for your body. In cold weather, it is often a challenge to leave hearth and home and venture into the wild. Outdoor exercise will increase your energy while decreasing tension, frustration, and depression, according to recent research published in *Environmental Science & Technology.*[xxi]

Some negative psychological effects may well be intensified in the winter, says adventure-fitness consultant Sean Burch, who set a world record running a marathon at the North Pole. "The heat and humidity in the summer can drag you down and tire you faster, but cold weather is invigorating," he says. "It stimulates your senses, tunes you in to your surroundings—it makes you feel alive."

There's a biological reason for that: All exercise increases your levels of feel-good hormones and neurotransmitters such as serotonin, dopamine, estrogen, and progesterone. Hormones and neurotransmitters modulate feelings of well-being, and lifestyle factors affect them, particularly if we are shut-ins during the long winter months. But because your body works harder in the cold, your hormone and neurotransmitter production is boosted even more, leading to a happier state of mind. Plus, exposure to natural light is a known depression fighter, especially for seasonal affective disorder, a condition caused by the shortened, dimmer days.

Bundle Up

Layer yourself and make sure your undergarments cover your stomach and hips. Try snow pants or long johns under your outer pants or running sweats. To counteract wind chill, you can add a scarf as face and neck protection. A couple of pairs of thermal or wool-blend socks, gloves, and a good cap are essential to complete your bundle. Lastly, make certain that your outerwear jacket is tested for cold, wind, and is waterproof.

Intelligent Warm Ups

Before you venture outside, walk indoors or jog in place for five minutes. When you head out, give your body time to adjust to the environment by taking short breaks every few minutes for the first 10 to 15 minutes. Don't push too hard too soon, but also don't stop for prolonged periods of time since your body temperature can dip faster in cold weather, increasing your risk of hypothermia.

Hydrate

You don't experience sweat losses in the winter like you do in the summer, so most people give minimal thought to staying hydrated. But you will still sweat just as much, especially if you're bundled up. If needed, try putting your water bottle under your layers to prevent it from freezing.

Timing is Everything

If the elements are severe, a midafternoon workout, when the temperatures are highest and the roads are clear, is a safer bet.

Best Winter Activities

Winter walking or running is great if you're properly geared and warmed up. Cross country skiing burns a ton of calories. Downhill skiing works hamstrings, quadriceps, and calf, hip, abdominal muscles, and foot muscles. Snowboarding works the same muscle groups as skiing and increases calorie burn. Ice skating is a good low-impact activity but Third and Fourth Generations beware: falling is dangerous and landing can cause loads of trauma. The same goes for ice hockey—leave this sport to the youth.

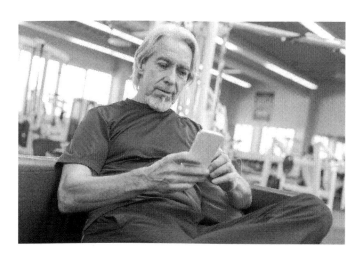

15   Fitness Tracking Technology

In the last 10 years or so, there's been a rapid rise in popularity for digital activity trackers. Most of these wearable devices wirelessly synchronize with a computer and smartphone app, recording your daily movements.

There are many reasons fitness trackers are popular: they give you feedback on numbers of steps, calories, distances, and in some cases heart rates and even sleep duration. You know what you've accomplished, and you know what you need to do to reach new goals.

Wearable technology will keep getting more accurate, allowing us to track more biometrics and get more feedback on fitness metrics so we can monitor progress. I expect that within a few years they will also provide health data that will help doctors monitor both diseases and wellness indicators.

In the meantime, today's trackers provide a way for everyone to take charge of their health and exercise, recording output (steps, distance covered, calories burned, food logs) and input (food and calories consumed), along with weight, heart rate, hydration, and sleep.

If you haven't tried one of these popular devices, I encourage you to start with one of the free apps for a smartphone. I think you'll find that it's fun to get feedback on your efforts. To find out more about wearable tech, use Google or any search engine. New devices are coming online all the time, so read the reviews and choose one that suits your needs.

My Fitbit

My personal experience using a Fitbit device for four years is that a step tracker has a positive effect on motivation. For example, if I know I took 10,000 steps yesterday (the American Heart Association's daily recommendation), I can decide to increase my goal the next day. And when I see that I recorded only 8,000 steps, I might decide to walk to the store instead of jumping in the car. Little motivational efforts add up and count for a lot.

Another reason trackers are fun is that they are social. I can share results with a friend and we can even compete. Most trackers allow you to connect with friends to view their data. This built-in social aspect makes the solitary work of fitness much more enjoyable.

While the numbers aren't 100 percent accurate, my latest device, the Fitbit Alta, a wrist model, has been tested at 90 percent accuracy. It also tells time and replaces the need for a watch.

The only thing more I'd wish to have in a tracker is an accurate heart rate reader. This doesn't have one, although other brands do. Reviewers are saying trackers aren't sufficiently accurate heart monitors when worn in a wrist band model. I use a heart rate app on my iPhone 6, but I know it isn't accurate either.

Experts say the only accurate heart rate monitors are the ones you wear around your chest. I'll wait until they come out with a more comfortable device. I've read that scientists are developing clothing and other means to record heart rate, sweat, and other health indicators.

The reason I would want a heart rate monitor is to know whether I am getting my heart rate up to

115 to 120 beats per minute while walking. That would be in the 65 to 75 percent range for my age. That is my target range for getting good cardiovascular benefits.

The accuracy isn't what matters. It is the knowledge that you get "credit" for your efforts. Psychologically, the record becomes a reward. For myself, I know that without an activity record, it would be easier to get discouraged on days when I don't want to do much.

Having iPhone or Fitbit tracking of days, weeks, and months of activities helps prevent discouragement and provides a bigger-picture perspective.

In the beginning months of acquiring a tracker, I got a little obsessed with the numbers, as did many of my friends. "How many steps did you do today?" we'd ask each other. If one of us forgot to wear our tracker, we were devastated, as if the exercise we were doing didn't count!

But what's a little obsession when it comes to exercise, right? Nobody is obsessed by the number of hours they spend watching TV, are they? Maybe they should be.

What trackers have taught me is that the time I spend reading and working on the computer can have a huge impact on my well-being. Although cerebral work is good for my brain fitness, my joints, muscles, and metabolism all stiffen up.

Our bodies were built to move, not sit. At least now I have a record of how much I'm moving around versus sitting. I've even taken to enjoying a bit of housework from time to time, as I get "credit" for the steps! Who knew Fitbit would make a better homemaker out of me?

What's interesting is to look at patterns over a whole week or month, or even a year. There's a perception that seniors fear technology and that we're challenged by computers, cellular phones, social media, and the like. If this is true for you, I humbly suggest you take some classes, or at the very least, seek an expert friend or a grandchild to guide you through any techno pitfalls.

Why is the understanding of high-tech devices relevant to your fitness and health goals? Today there is a virtual plethora of free exercise charts, calorie-counters, and medical, health, and diet applications (apps) you can download to your computer, your iPad, and your smartphone.

Tech Wearables: Why They Help You

Even if you're the poster boy for *Computing for Dummies*, check out some of the fitness gadgets and apps. Wearable technology is here, and it is fun as well as utilitarian. Wearables make technology easy by interweaving electronics, software, sensors and connectivity into wristbands, watches, headbands, scales, eyewear, and even sports equipment, enabling objects to exchange and record data.

Many seniors are wearing activity trackers and have a smartphone in their pocket, both of which are gathering motion-sensing data through the accelerometer and gyroscope inside. Add to this a multitude of biometrics such as tracking blood pressure, REM sleep, heart monitoring, and reminders of when you've been sitting at the computer too long, and you'll understand why we're joining the technology era.

Many of these apps can be a boon to get you started, keep you involved, and provide you with training exercises specific to your age, sport, and short- and long-term goals. Patsi is a big fan of Fitbit tracking devices, but there are many other brands that are fun, useful, and motivating.

As a bit of a hardware geek, I believe there may be better wearable tech products coming out soon. Alternatively, check out products from Jawbone and Garmin Connect.

Never before have computing devices been small enough to be worn relatively comfortably on the body around the clock, presenting opportunities for breakthrough medical and fitness tracking.

The nerd in me can see a day, perhaps in the very near future, when small, virtually undetectable sensors will be sewn/woven (or 3D printed) into our apparel with the intention of "communicating" with multiple smart devices. One day you may walk into your home, where the front door will recognize you and open automatically, the central air conditioning will sense your body temperature and turn on the heating or cooling, and your smart refrigerator will diagnose your need for hydration and automatically dispense a glass of ice water.

Biometrics is the measurement and statistical analysis of people's physical and behavioral characteristics. Your most vital biometrics, such as heart rate, rhythm, and pressure, can be monitored by these wearable sensors, and one day soon, your clothing or watch will remotely alert a healthcare monitoring system and your doctor as to your condition.

How we wear or carry our technology continues to evolve, as mobile devices themselves change. It's when these devices disappear into our clothing that a change occurs in our relationship to the technologies we use. Wearable tech could have a huge impact on senior health, fitness and safety soon.

App Alternatives

I like the fitness apps from FitnessBuilder.com. The site offers a free download of hundreds of exercise routines for your iPhone, iPad, or Android phone. There are visuals with systematic instructions for a multitude of sports and fitness routines. For example, there are exercise routines for:

- Abs and Core
- 10-minute Energy Booster
- Balance and Stability
- Best Butt Exercises
- Cycling Conditioning
- Golf Conditioning
- Hiking Training
- Pilates
- Senior Workout
- Stretching
- Tennis Conditioning
- Travel Conditioning
- Yoga De-stress

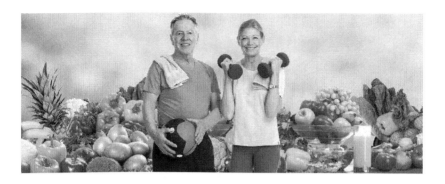

16   Food and Fat

Seniors develop allergies over the years and become sensitive to specific foods, on top of all the airborne particles. Two that come to mind are gluten (the protein in wheat, rye, and barley) and lactose (the sugar in milk). If you have a food allergy, you'll know it—immediate digestive distress. But many of us have a sensitivity that goes undiagnosed and can lead to lethargy, water retention, gas, and of course cortisol elevation and fat accumulation. If you suspect this, try cutting out things like wheat and dairy for a few weeks and see how your body responds.

Besides storing excess calories, one of the physiological purposes for body fat is to store toxins. When you take in a lot of toxins through the environment or from processed foods, they get stored in fat deposits, especially around the liver and pancreas—in belly fat.

How can you reduce toxin exposure? Buy organic produce (regular produce is often sprayed with pesticides that act as toxins in our body). Cut back on alcohol, which the body treats as a toxin. Reduce consumption of processed foods—I can't help but think that all those chemicals, preservatives, and artificial sweeteners are perceived as toxins in the body. And finally, eat more detoxifying foods (and not some BS detox plan designed to sell you 100 different supplements). I mean real foods that naturally serve as detoxifiers—i.e., organic vegetables and herbs such as peppermint, eucalyptus, cilantro, wormwood, black walnut, and dandelion.

Note: Eucalyptus dried leaves and oil are natural remedies used to make medicine believed to combat bacteria and fungi, pain and inflammation and block chemicals that cause asthma. Wormwood can be consumed many different ways, but the most typical and effective way to get results is by drinking it in a tea or consuming it by tincture; but for no longer than four weeks at a time.

My wife is a coffee lover, and the research is quite clear that too much caffeine elevates levels of cortisol, the stress hormone. Moderate amounts do not have detrimental effects on the central nervous system and can assist in the fat loss process by increasing lipolysis and acting as a thermogenic aid. But too much coffee can cause sleep problems, plus dizziness, diarrhea, increased thirst, headache, fever and irritability.

According to the Mayo Clinic, the recommended amount of caffeine is 400 milligrams per day for healthy adults. Considering that one 12 oz. serving of black coffee contains 240 mg and additionally chocolate, soft drinks, some medicines, some chewing gums and all energy drinks (Red Bull contains 80 mg caffeine), let the buyer beware.

If you are eating crap, not getting quality energy from real food, not sleeping well, and using caffeine and energy drinks to compensate (drinking a large Starbucks coffee, plus five Red Bulls and six diet sodas a day), well, you see where that might lead to problems. And if you are using coffee as a vessel for sugar and cream, consider that you don't really like coffee —you like sugar and cream.

The 85 Percent Rule

Now I know some of you are thinking, *Rob's crazy and I'm not cutting out all of that. I must live my life.*

Well, I get it. But my aim is to present the absolute ideal scenario. In reality, it's up to you to find your own compromises. What has worked well for most of my friends is to follow the 85 percent rule. Follow the ideal path 85 percent of the time, and 15 percent of the time, do whatever you want. If you do that, you will be just fine. Imagine what cutting out all sugar 85 percent of the time could do for your body and health.

Be aware that many of these "habits" are unrecognized addictions. Can you live your life without caffeine? Are you addicted to sugar? What's going on inside your neural pathways?

We are a generation of pseudo-addicts. We live for feel good quick fixes and instant gratification.

We've spawned whole industries that greedily cater to our dependencies, like the fast food, tobacco, caffeine, sugar, and pharmaceutical industries, who have built empires while addicting us to their products. Those short bursts of pleasure that make us feel (chemically) better about ourselves and our crazy world don't seem to bother us much in our third, fourth and fifth decades, but when we hit the senior years—watch out!

One way of altering any addiction is to rewire neural pathways and substitute dependencies for an exercise and fitness "fix." In a very short time, you can experience the highs of natural dopamine and endorphins created by vigorous exercise, which can

eventually replace any of the other addictions
mentioned above.

Belly Fat

Two of the most abundant compounds in the
average modern American diet are two of the worst
ingredients for cellular health—concentrated fructose
and trans fats. Both compounds have been researched
and proven to be linked to many of our most
troublesome diseases, as well as insulin resistance and
abdominal obesity.

To avoid both these dangerous ingredients,
simply "stop eating crap." Try to reduce trans-
unsaturated fatty acids (trans fats come mostly from
packaged snack foods, fried foods, anything with
hydrogenated oil or margarine). Cut out concentrated
sources of fructose: high fructose corn syrup (which is
technically one molecule of glucose plus one molecule
of fructose), cane sugar, packaged fruit juices and
dried fruits, and many foods that are marketed as
"healthy" yet contain just as much sugar, if not more,
than table sugar. Fructose should be consumed in
much smaller amounts than in the average American
diet, and in the way in which Mother Nature
intended—via seasonal whole fruit.

If you stick to this first principle alone, that
should take care of about 90 percent of the problem.

Almost everything else related to belly fat accumulation can be attributed to the hormone cortisol which is released when we experience stress. And while cortisol is a necessary and integral part of normal functioning, problems (including that damn belly fat) can arise with chronic cortisol overproduction.

The Fit-Everywhere-Else-But-Fat-on-the-Belly Syndrome

I'm seeing this syndrome increasingly in gyms these days, as super low-carb diets designed for the sick, sedentary population are being adopted by fit athletes engaging in intense anaerobic training. Remember what I said about different diets being more appropriate for different demographics? The athlete's training creates a unique physiological and metabolic environment much different than for more sedentary people.

Here's the thing. Strength training puts a unique stress on the body; it creates cellular damage, better known as inflammation, that demands repair, and it depletes muscle glycogen stores. A heavy workout, such as an hour of weight training, must be offset by proper nutritional intake. This will ultimately lead our bodies to an adaptive response—strength, energy, muscle gain, metabolic boost, and whoopee--belly fat loss.

184

This is not happening in today's carbo-phobic fad diets. With no carbs in response to training, the body remains in a constant catabolic state where cortisol is the dominant hormone. Consequently, you get no muscle growth; instead, the body uses lean muscle tissue as fuel. Furthermore, when cortisol levels remain elevated, it leads to fat accumulation around the midsection. Guys and gals who are consistently training hard, following the low-carb dietary trend, thinking they are doing everything right, are lean everywhere else, but have a layer of flab hanging around their belt line.

Insulin is a misinterpreted hormone these days in the low-carb fad diets. No hormone your body produces naturally is inherently bad; it just needs to be controlled. The chronic elevation or overproduction of insulin will lead to fat gain. But in the right amounts and situations (following an intense workout where insulin sensitivity is high), itcan be a good thing.

If this resonates with you, my best advice is adding some non-fructose, non-gluten containing carbs back into your diet (potatoes, sweet potatoes, brown rice) to reduce belly fat. At the very least, start with a protein drink in the post-workout window (45 minutes post training). If you work out hard, keep your protein to carb ratio around 1:1. If you consume 20g of protein and eat 20g of starchy carbs per meal.

So, all this resistance training requires a balanced diet of both protein and carbohydrates, contrary to many of the food fads you may read. A body in motion cannot survive in an unhealthy state living off protein only or carbs only.

It is scary to think of all the fad diets that find their way into our kitchens every year. The next time you think of embarking on a fad diet, you need to ask yourself why so many of them exist in the first place. Surely if any of these diets worked, the other pseudoscience diet fascists would have stopped their evil schemes long ago.

By the way, the same goes for that crazy get-fit-quick scheme: as seen on TV workout contraptions. If you believe in fad diets and aerobic contrivances, I have some nice costume jewelry I'd like to sell you.

"Back to the Future..."

I remember when families cooked with real butter, ice cream came from whole milk, and when we didn't eat our veggies we were lectured about the starving kids in China. Add to that there were no GMO foods and no DDT pesticides. We could walk barefoot on grass without getting sick from pesticide-laden garden pollutants such as, herbicides, insecticides, and fertilizers.

Yes, I spent my entire youth in the sun, sans SPF, soaking up freckles and vitamin D.

Our produce and meats were free range, our salmon came from Alaska and shrimp were harvested from the sea. As early as 1962 we began to realize that DDT was poisoning wildlife, the environment, and endangering human health, and the public protest launched a modern environmental movement in the United States; DDT was banned (could that occur in today's culture of corporate corruption?).

As seniors, we have been exposed repeatedly to these unfortunate, deregulated, and man-made hazards in our environment...and yet we are still here. But what, if anything, are we doing about this assault on our health and wellbeing?

PATSI SAYS

Fat for Fuel

I don't always agree with Rob on diet. While what he says is true, and it works for him, my own experience with the ketogenic diet has been positive. This regimen advises low net carbohydrates, moderate protein, and high fat. After two to four weeks, metabolism switches from burning glucose to burning fat for fuel.

I've always eaten relatively low-calorie meals, few carbohydrates, and low fat. This explains why, after a year of resistance training and trying to build muscles, my body fat percentage barely dropped. Instead of growing muscle, my body used muscle for fuel. Not enough protein in my diet, too much sugar, and hardly any fat.

The solution is to add more protein to my diet, eliminate sugar, wheat, pasta, and unnecessary carbs, and start eating the right kinds of fat that the body can burn as fuel: saturated fats, in particular. When I did this, my body fat dropped from 28% to 26% and muscle increased—finally!

This isn't new and isn't a fad diet. Research has shown how switching to fat for fuel not only is healthy, but is recommended for people with cancer, seizures, and other chronic diseases. It promotes mitochondrial health, reduces oxidative stress and inflammation, and delays aging. Athletes find they can prolong training and recover quickly. Best of all, when the body switches to burning fat for fuel, the brain thrives.

I'm still learning how to prepare meals that contain high fat and moderate protein, and there are plenty of websites online with great and easy recipes (look for ketogenic diets). In the appendixes, I recommend a couple of books to explain the science behind this revolutionary approach to eating healthfully. So far, simply by eliminating wheat and sugar, my gut is happier, my brain fog has lifted, and meals are way more delicious and satisfying.

It's up to every senior to find a diet that works for him or her and which is satisfying and appeals to the palate, the digestive system, and energy levels, and is beneficial to their new exercise regimen.

Hidden Dangers of Belly Fat

According to an article on the MSN health and fitness site, the issue isn't losing weight, but rather reducing the invisible fat found around the middle of the body, or visceral fat.[1]

Where you carry your body weight says a lot about your health. Those who retain weight around the midsection ("apple-shaped" people) tend to be at higher risk for disease than those who retain weight at the hips ("pear-shaped" people).

Body-fat percentage: for a rough approximation of acceptable body-fat percentage, calculate your waist-to-hip ratio. For men, the ratio should be no higher than 0.90, for women, no higher than 0.83.

189

For people who fall outside of the normal body-fat range, getting enough exercise is crucial for addressing visceral fat, the type of fat that you can't necessarily see and that collects around your organs, increasing your risk for disease.

"Exercise disproportionately targets visceral fat," Gary R. Hunter, a professor of human studies at the University of Alabama at Birmingham, told the *New York Times* in 2015.[2] Research bears this out. A 2010 study published in the journal *Obesity* found that sedentary women who began a moderate exercise regimen lost 10 percent of their visceral fat during the year-long study program.[3]

Falls and Fractures

As women age, we become more vulnerable to falls and fractures. After menopause, we lose bone density, balance, and flexibility. When we take a misstep and start to fall, it's harder to catch ourselves, stop the fall, or come out of it intact. Our bones break more easily than before.

Many health sites on the Internet will tell you about the appalling loss of quality of life that happens after a serious fall. The dangers of falls and fractures are not just to women in their 80s and 90s. It can happen any time, especially if you start letting your body deteriorate. That is something you can fight against. You can take an active stance and lower the risk of fractures by exercising.

Did you know one of the most serious fall injuries is a broken hip? It is hard to recover from a hip fracture, and afterward, many people are not able to live on their own. As the population gets older, the number of hip fractures is likely to go up. In the U.S. alone:

- Each year at least 250,000 older people—those 65 and older—are hospitalized for hip fractures.
- More than 95 percent of hip fractures are caused by falling, usually by falling sideways.
- Women experience 75 percent of all hip fractures.
- Women fall more often than men.
- Women are more susceptible to osteoporosis, a disease that weakens bones and makes them more likely to break.

We're not alone when we recommend weight-bearing exercise to prevent osteoporosis. No matter what other activities you do—sports, swimming, dancing, yoga—you should include some strength training with free weights or body resistance. You'll be glad you did the next time you start to slip and fall.

Fifteen years ago, I had a bone density scan that indicated osteopenia, the precursor to osteoporosis. This year, my scan was in the normal range. I attribute the improvement to my strength-training regimen.

Most Seniors Are Sedentary

A National Center for Health Statistics survey in 1995 showed that only about 25 percent of older Americans exercise regularly. Another study showed that 58 percent of older Americans believe they get as much exercise as they need.

Now think about it: if only a fourth of seniors exercise regularly but over half believe they do, it doesn't add up. This could be explained by faulty thinking. It's a common mental bias to believe we are better off than we are and that we are "just fine." While a good self-image is important, crossing over into denial puts our health at risk.

We aren't motivated to exercise just for the sake of exercising because it isn't programmed into our genes. Running is, hunting prey is, killing animals for lunch—all these activities provided a serious advantage to our gene pool. In the natural selection process, only the fit survived to reproduce and perpetuate the race.

And while being fit is vital, going to a gym just for the fun of it is not. In fact, we are programmed to

conserve energy when not in danger of being eaten
alive.

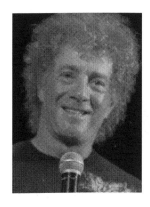 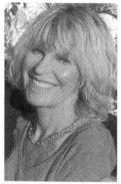

17 Why Should Anyone Listen to Us?

Admittedly, we are not longevity specialists, medical doctors, nutritionists, or physical exercise trainers. You should know that we're not giving anyone individual advice, and just because we do something doesn't mean you should. Everyone's different, and even more so when it comes to seniors.

We've researched and investigated the facts surrounding aging and fitness; however, much of our advice on healthy living practices are based on our own opinions and experiences as well as those of other active seniors we have interviewed.

At age 38, I was overweight, perpetually tired, stressed out, quick to anger, prone to common colds, and yes, my body was beginning to die. The brain begins to age as early as age 20. And as we get older, the number of nerve cells—or neurons—in the brain decreases. We start with around 100 billion, but in our 20s this number begins to decline. By age 38, I was probably losing up to 10,000 per day, affecting memory, co-ordination, and brain function. Besides the brain, at 38 years old, other important organs began to decline, including lungs, vision, heart, muscles, teeth, skin, and hair.

To say that I have reversed the aging process for my organs would be a stretch. Allow me, though, to say that today, at 77, I am in better shape-- physically, mentally, and emotionally--than I was at half my age. And indeed, I still have my hair!

PATSI SAYS

Our main objective for writing this book is to help people entering the "third half" of life to adopt exercise and fitness to prevent diseases that attack the body and mind. While physical fitness can be recuperated after disease and healing, it makes sense that preventing chronic diseases in the first place should be every senior's objective. And that notion goes well beyond seniors.

As for Rob, he's been extremely physically active his whole life, so two hours of tennis and an hour in the gym is not unusual. And yes, there are days when he doesn't feel like it and a few when he's so tired afterward that he doesn't do much else. Nevertheless, we do something, whatever we can, and try to make it fun. And it's paying off.

Here's what we know:

- You don't have to be a lifelong athlete to adopt a healthy exercise habit.
- If you aren't using your muscles, you are losing your muscles... and brain cells.
- Anyone can and should start at a comfortable level and build up.
- You start now, do a little bit on two, then three, then four to six days a week, and you keep accumulating health benefits.
- You make it fun and social by playing sports or training with friends.
- If you maintain more healthy than unhealthy days, you will get fit, be happy, and live longer.
- All exercise requires healthy (real) food for the body and brain, and one without the other doesn't work.

We encourage you to reject those awful cultural biases that paint seniors as weak, sick, and irrelevant.

Many of us are finally free of the many responsibilities that consumed our time, focus, and energy for decades, such as raising our families and having full-time careers. This truly can be your golden age where you are more creative, alive, and thriving than ever before.

Sometimes extreme measures are needed.

Rob and I decided more than a couple of decades ago to go all out for health. We don't smoke, don't drink any alcohol, and the only drugs we use we buy at Walgreen's. But we're not saints, and it's up to you to make those lifestyle choices.

Rob has a serious heart condition, I have mild arrhythmia, and we've got the seniors' medley of bad body parts and surgeries (knees, back, shoulders).

When it comes to life, nobody gets out alive. But there are some better ways to experience this whole old-age adventure. If you make life fun and adventuresome, some of the pain gets ignored. AND, here's one big secret: exercise reduces a lot of the causes of pain in joints and muscles.

What we're doing is works for us. Exercise has been documented by medical experts as the only recommended solution to actually REVERSE the aging process: physical exercise will preserve your health and keep your body from weakening and getting sick as you age.

Appendix 1: What's in a Brain?

The brain accounts for about two percent of your body weight, but consumes 20 percent of the energy available to you. It's composed of 60 percent fat, which is why consuming healthy fats is especially important for your brain (avocados, salmon, fish, and fish oil supplements).

Both EPA and DHA are components of omega-3 fats found in fish and they are used in brain tissue. A major accelerator of brain aging is chronic inflammation (over-activation of the immune system). That is why we need to avoid eating high-glycemic-index carbohydrates such as sugary foods and starches.

Brain Supplements

Vinpocetine is a natural supplement derived from the periwinkle plant which increases blood flow to the brain and increases production of ATP (adenosine triphosphate), the brain's energy source. It has been shown to enhance memory for people with both normal and impaired memory. You can find it in health food stores as it's not a medicine.

Alzheimer's disease is an irreversible, progressive brain disorder that slowly destroys memory and thinking skills, and eventually the ability to carry out the simplest tasks. In most people with Alzheimer's, symptoms first appear in their mid-60s. Estimates vary, but experts suggest that more than 5 million Americans may have Alzheimer's at any given time.

Alzheimer's disease is currently ranked as the sixth leading cause of death in the United States, but recent estimates indicate that the disorder may rank third, just behind heart disease and cancer, as a cause of death for older people.

Alzheimer's is the most common cause of dementia among older adults. Dementia is the term that encompasses general loss of cognitive functioning—thinking, remembering, and reasoning—and of behavioral abilities to such an extent that it interferes with a person's daily life and activities.

Alzheimer's disease is complex, and it is unlikely that any one drug or other intervention can successfully treat it. Current approaches focus on helping people maintain mental function, manage behavioral symptoms, and slow or delay the symptoms of disease. Researchers hope to develop therapies targeting specific genetic, molecular, and cellular mechanisms so that the actual underlying cause of the disease can be stopped or prevented.

From what I hear from our senior friends, the thing they fear most is Alzheimer's or dementia. With the first sign of forgetting someone's name, we joke about "senior moments" and "sometimer's disease." Everyone fears losing memory and the ability to enjoy life.

Many seniors have had to take care of parents or grandparents with Alzheimer's. Here's what the research explains, according to the National Institute on Aging.

Some 5.2 million people in the U.S. had Alzheimer's in 2014, a number that is expected to triple by 2050. While scientists are still struggling to find causes and cures, there are several reports of high functioning seniors who were discovered to have had Alzheimer's only by a post-mortem autopsy. They had no symptoms at all and died from other causes.

In these cases, these seniors had active lifestyles and high cognitive functioning beyond what was expected for their age despite what should have been debilitating plaque in their brains. Scientists conclude that some people with abundant cognitive reserves can slow or delay symptoms of Alzheimer's and brain dysfunction.[1]

Cognitive Reserves

What are cognitive reserves? Here's what the National Institute of Health reports in a study by Yaakof Stern published in *Lancet Neurology* in 2012. **Cognitive Reserves in Aging and Alzheimer's disease:**

The concept of reserve accounts for individual differences in susceptibility to age-related brain changes or Alzheimer's disease-related pathology.

There is evidence that some people can tolerate more of these changes than others and still maintain function. Epidemiological studies suggest that lifetime exposures, including educational and occupational attainment, and leisure activities in late life, can increase this reserve.

For example, there is a reduced risk of developing Alzheimer's disease in individuals with higher educational or occupational attainment. It is convenient to think of two types of reserves: brain reserve, which refers to actual differences in the brain itself that may increase tolerance of pathology, and cognitive reserves.

"Cognitive reserves" refers to individual differences in how tasks are performed that may allow some people to be more resilient than others. The concept of cognitive reserves holds out the promise of interventions that could slow cognitive aging or reduce the risk of dementia.

There is clear evidence that mental and physical fitness can delay the onset of symptoms of brain dysfunction. First, let's talk about the effects of physical exercise on cognitive functions.

The neurobiological effects of physical exercise involve a wide range of interrelated effects on brain structure, brain function, and cognition. A large body of research in humans has demonstrated that consistent aerobic exercise (30 minutes every day) induces persistent beneficial behavioral and neural plasticity as well as healthy alterations in gene expression in the brain.

Some of these long-term effects include increased neuron growth, increased neurological activity (signaling), improved coping with stress, enhanced cognitive control of behavior, improved memory, and structural and functional improvements in the brain.

The effects of exercise on cognition have important implications for improving productivity, preserving cognitive function in old age, preventing or treating certain neurological disorders, and improving overall quality of life.[2]

How Can Walking Improve the Brain?

If your 30-minute walk gets your heart rate up in the aerobic exercise ranges of 60 to 70 percent of your maximum rate, you've halted some of the brain decay of aging. Most people will need to walk very fast to do that, or walk for a longer period.

In one study of previously sedentary seniors, one group walked 30 minutes every day for 12 months. Another spent 30 minutes daily in the gym doing stretching exercises. At the end of 12 months they were examined with blood tests, cognitive testing, and brain imaging. Only the group of seniors who walked showed positive improvements, including growth of new brain cells.

Aerobic Exercise Grows New Brain Cells

(Excerpts from NPR "Aerobic Exercise May Improve Memory in Seniors" February 21, 2011)

Neuroscientist Peter Snyder, a researcher at Brown University's Alpert Medical School and Rhode Island Hospital, says the hippocampus is one of those brain areas that continues to form new cells and make new connections between cells. (The hippocampus is a crucial area of the brain involved in memory and learning.)

"What we're finding is that of all of these noninvasive ways of intervening, it is exercise that seems to have the most efficacy at this point—more so than nutritional supplements, vitamins, and cognitive interventions," says Snyder, who studies what we can do to maintain memory as our brains age.[3]

Some of the most provocative evidence on the power of exercise on the brain comes from a study published in the National Academy of Sciences by neuroscientist Art Kramer at the University of Illinois at Urbana-Champaign. Kramer and his colleagues have documented the impact of exercise on the growth of the hippocampus in a small group of elderly people over the course of one year.

"The participants in our study were 120 very sedentary people," Kramer says. All the participants in the study had MRI brain scans done before the study began and again a year later when the study ended. Then the researchers analyzed the MRI data.

"What we found," Kramer says, "was that individuals in the aerobic group showed increases in the volume of their hippocampus. "The increase in volume— again for the aerobic but not for the non-aerobic group—was about 2 percent. "The 2 percent increase we can think of as turning back the clock about two years," Kramer says. By comparison, "the individuals in the control group — in the toning and stretching group — lost about 1.5 percent [of their hippocampal volume], so we can think of it as about a 3.5 percent difference compared to those individuals who didn't benefit aerobically."[4]

The evidence that exercise is good for the brain isn't limited to seniors, of course. But it is more significant because it will counteract the decaying processes which accelerate as one gets older. Even if only a small percentage of new brain cells grow after exercise, it makes a huge difference to older people who normally would be losing cells regularly.

Exercise-induced Brain Growth

One of the most significant effects of exercise on the brain is the increased synthesis and expression of BDNF, which stands for "brain derived neurotropic factor" (neurotropic means it grows new brains cells). This neuropeptide hormone travels from muscles and crosses the blood/brain barrier to stimulate growth and efficiency of cognitive functions.

Exercise causes increases in brain BDNF signaling, associated with beneficial changes that improve cognitive function, mood, and memory. Furthermore, research has provided a great deal of support for the role of BDNF in growing new hippocampal neurons, synaptic plasticity, and neural repair.

Engaging in moderate-to-high intensity aerobic exercise such as running, swimming, and cycling, increases BDNF biosynthesis through myokine signaling, resulting in up to a threefold increase in blood plasma and brain BDNF levels.

Exercise intensity is positively correlated with the magnitude of increased BDNF biosynthesis and expression.

Exercise Grows Brain Cells in Just Three Months

Two reviews of randomized controlled trials with durations of three to 12 months have examined the effects of physical exercise on the characteristics of Alzheimer's disease. The reviews found beneficial effects of physical exercise on cognitive function, the rate of cognitive decline, and the ability to perform activities of daily living in individuals with Alzheimer's disease. One review suggested that, based upon transgenic mouse models, the cognitive effects of exercise on Alzheimer's disease may result from a reduction in the quantity of amyloid plaque.

It may seem obvious that exercise would be good for the brain as well as the body, since exercise speeds up transportation of oxygen to the blood and means more oxygen and energy get delivered to the brain. But the beneficial processes involve more than just oxygen. Neuropeptide hormones such as BDNG, IGF-1, and VEGF pass the blood/brain barrier. These substances are called signaling hormones, sending stimulating messages to improve brain function, including growth of new cells.

Continuous exercise can produce short-term euphoria, an affective state associated with feelings of profound contentment, elation, and well-being, which is colloquially known as "runner's high" in distance running or "rower's high" in rowing. Current medical reviews indicate that several endogenous euphoriants are responsible for producing exercise-related euphoria.

Think about that the next time you say, "I'm too tired to exercise!" Exercise will deliver your body's naturally occurring feel-good hormones right to your brain's door—no charge.

You don't have to be a brain scientist or understand what happens on a cellular level. Just trust that getting off the couch or out of your car will provoke energy, pain relief, and healing substances all the way down to your mitochondria.

Just move it. The good vibrations will kick in.

Mental Workouts for Brain Fitness

The business of brain health products totals over a billion dollars a year and keeps growing. The popularity of games for the brain isn't accounted for by any scientific evidence that they work, but rather by our fascination with mental puzzles.

According to a 2013 article in *Forbes*, brain products are big business.

All over the marketplace, entrepreneurs are hopping on the brain health bandwagon. Whether it's software that promises to improve your memory, games that claim to fend off dementia, supplements or foods that fuel brain power, or self-help books and gurus showing how to enhance cognitive function, there's been an explosion of investment in brain fitness.

According to a study by SharpBrains, the market for brain health software alone grew from $600 million in annual revenues in 2009 to more than one billion dollars by the end of 2012. The researchers forecast this market to reach four to 10 billion dollars by 2020, with six billion being the most likely scenario.[5]

The hype is seductive. One author who claims to be a brain expert suggests that, "You don't have to take a pill or watch a DVD or buy a product to enhance your mental performance. Your mind can be strengthened just like a muscle, and it only takes 100 seconds a day."

He presents a five-step meditative exercise to build a positive self-image, concluding, "Just as your body responds to consistent strength training, your mind responds to regular mental workouts."

Oh boy, in just a minute and a half, great! Wait, though, there's no secret here. We've known about the positive effect of meditation and affirmations for a long time. No one is disputing this common-sense approach to reinforcing a healthy frame of mind.

But it is a big leap to say you can change your brain or strengthen your mind permanently in a minute and a half. I mention this article because it is an example of how misleading some publications can be when it comes to anything about the brain.

Beware of brain buzz. Not all you read about the brain is based on solid information. To date, the only proven program to improve brain function is physical exercise. (What? Did you think you could do it sitting on your butt in front of the computer?)

Mental games are good for the brain anyway; they're just not going to replace the need for exercise. Some exercises are better than others for building a better brain.

Those activities requiring multiple movements at the same time are challenging for the brain and contribute to maintaining and growing neurons. For example, dancing requires learning steps, pacing, patterns, and multiple simultaneous body movements. So does tennis, ping-pong, and golf—or most any sport, for that matter. Playing the piano, learning to play a musical instrument, learning a language—these are all especially good for the brain.

Word and math games will keep your mental retrieval skills sharp. Some complex computer games involving multiple players, story simulations, and strategies are great for maintaining brain strength.

All mental activities, but especially challenging ones, are good for the brain and, in that sense, similar to engaging your muscles. Use it or lose it. But the key is to have stretch goals, for both your body and your brain.

The Future of Brain Technology

In the next couple of decades, scientists envision injecting nanobots into the brain through capillaries. The nanobots will interact with your biological neurons to provide an extension to your brain. In this way, your brain, aided by nanobots, will experience total immersion in any virtual reality you request.

Operating from within your own nervous system, and perhaps accessing information from cloud systems, you will be able to expand your memory and thinking ability. Far off in the future? This is predicted for the 2030s by authors Kurzweil and Grossman, in their book *Transcend*.[6]

Taking out the garbage every day uses your muscles, but doesn't challenge them to grow unless you have more progressively heavier garbage each day.

Meditating regularly is great for relieving stress, anxiety, and tension and does wonderful things on multiple levels. But it doesn't grow new brain cells. Jigsaw puzzles, Sudoku, and all the expensive (or free) computer games and software are fun, sometimes challenging, but won't guarantee a better brain.

Why? Because to grow new brain cells, you need certain biochemical hormones (BDNF, IGF-1, and VEGF) and these are produced through exercise in the muscles and sent to the brain as a signal to grow.

Bonus Gifts for Our Readers

10 Mistakes Healthy Seniors Make
(...and their consequences in 5-10 years)

You may think you're doing okay because you're still healthy.
The habits you have today will determine if you thrive as a
senior... or barely survive.

For this report and other special gifts to our readers, visit our
private page:

www.seniorfitness4life.com/thanks-enlisting-war-aging/

Appendix 2: The Stories

Case Study: Linda

Linda wakes up from six hours of restless sleep. She is stiff, sore, and more tired than when she went to bed. She sits on the edge of her bed and tries to plan her day. In a few minutes, she collapses on the bed and stretches her arms, legs, and back. It is with herculean effort that she finally rises, makes her way to the bathroom, and brushes her teeth.

This is a typical morning for Linda since she retired last year. She shuffles into her kitchen, turns on the countertop TV, prepares a breakfast consisting of coffee and a buttered bagel, and watches the local news.

After her morning shower, she dresses in her lounging sweat suit, rests on her balcony, and reads the morning paper. She mulls over several articles regarding retiree wellness and an ad from a local health club. That's about as close as Linda wants to come to exercise—hefting the paper in a sporty outfit.

Linda piddles around the house the remainder of the morning, tidying and chatting on her mobile phone, until it's time to meet some friends for their tri-weekly luncheon. She changes into a more fashionable and looser-fitting fleece sweat suit and drives her car the five blocks to the restaurant.

There is no parking available. Linda, ever aware of her fixed income, nevertheless opts for valet parking service and walks stiffly into the restaurant and embraces her three friends.

Linda thinks she is scrupulous about her diet and orders a luncheon salad, and unfortunately, buttermilk ranch dressing with 160 calories, 17 g fat and 280 mg sodium. Her beverage of choice is the house iced tea, to which she adds two packets or 20g of pure sugar. Based on what Linda believes, she has just consumed a heart-healthy lunch, so she rewards herself with Brownie Sundae Cheesecake, adding another 1,368 calories, 61 grams of fat, and 580 milligrams of sodium to her "sensible" lunch.

She had no intention to be unhealthy and denies that at age 51 she might be aging badly. Linda returns home, stuffed, lethargic and drained from her meal. She loosens the drawstring on her sweatpants and lies flat on the bed. She awakens two and a half hours later. Her back and legs ache. She heads to the kitchen and pops three ibuprofen tablets into her mouth. She turns on the TV, eats a bag of chips, washes them down with a diet soda and watches cooking shows and sitcoms until dinner time.

215

Linda had plans to cook herself a healthy dinner, but when she arrives in the kitchen she realizes that she is far too tired to keep that promise. Her feet hurt as she stands by the stove and warms her dinner of canned soup, bread and butter, and some left-over chicken.

Linda eats part of her dinner standing in the kitchen and the other half in front of the TV. She watches TV for another hour and then retreats to the kitchen to reward herself with a bowl of ice cream. She watches TV until she falls asleep and the TV awakens her. Then she drags her weary body to bed for another night of tossing and turning.

Before she falls asleep she makes a mental note to get some exercise tomorrow and eat better. For a fleeting moment, she realizes she might be aging badly, but then focuses on her healthy intentions for tomorrow.

Linda is neither stupid nor lazy. She, like so many of you, is caught in a difficult spiral that many retirees and Third Agers experience. Linda believes that her early retirement is an excuse to rest and, in her case, to do as little as possible.

Intellectually, Linda knows that she should eat better and get out of the house and exercise, but she lacks motivation to change her life patterns and get started. She did not intend to live this way, but on her fixed retirement income her plans to travel, eat organic foods, join a gym, and improve her mind have not materialized, and she is headed toward a deep depression and potential diseases of the body and mind.

Linda finds new excuses every day that support her current unhealthy habits; excuses that allow her to eat crap and waste her life watching television. It prevents her from exercising and causes her to lose valuable sleep. With only a few minor lifestyle changes, Linda could be on her way to a long health span and a happier, more fulfilled life.

Julie's Story

I hadn't seen Julie for 15 years. We'd studied business coaching together and enjoyed a few tennis games when I was living in San Diego. Julie is a successful coach and consultant who's always had healthy habits. We reconnected by taking a two-hour walk around beautiful Mission Bay and Beach.

"I'm really angry! I'm 61 and suddenly, I'm hit with weird things like high cholesterol and other health challenges. I've always exercised, don't eat junk, I'm a healthy person, I don't get sick! Ever. I hardly ever see a doctor. What's going on?"

I smiled because I remembered 10 years ago. The only pills I took when I was Julie's age were vitamins. From that age on, each year came with new prescriptions—and I was healthy! But between 61 and 65, I had a major incident of heart fibrillation, shingles, back surgery, cataract surgery, and a breast cancer scare.

I was tempted to remind Julie that she wasn't 30 or 40 but kept my mouth shut. She knew the answer to her question; she knew that she was starting to age. Like me, she never really thought it would happen to her because she was already doing more than what was recommended to stay healthy and disease-free.

Julie's situation is common among smart individuals who practice sports and healthy habits most of their lives. Signs of aging often come gradually, gently, and unobtrusively: a few skin changes, slower reaction time, less balance, gradual weight gain, and less energy. Occasionally we can't remember a name as quickly as before. But sometimes, as in Julie's case, symptoms strike in groups and suddenly.

Then, this past summer, Julie noticed changing health indicators: her cholesterol levels rose from 215 to 285 and the doctor was recommending Lipitor, a statin drug with side effects. Her thyroid levels required medication. And she was dealing with a ringing in her ears.

For the first time in her life, Julie felt like she was losing control of her health. And because of her strong personality traits, this wasn't something she found easy to just "breathe into."

I can totally relate to this feeling. My own feelings of helplessness over health occurred when I reached the age range when my first-degree family members all died. You may feel as if you have reached your own point of no return.

Case Study: Sally

- Sally M., a 69-year-old female, weight 160 lbs. and height 5'7", with a BMI of 25.1 (normal)
- Had not exercised in years except for yoga and stretching classes
- Had never used any type of exercise equipment (e.g., treadmill, bike)
- Very high cholesterol and blood pressure (currently on meds)
- At high risk for obesity, osteoporosis, arthritis, and diabetes
- Bone density measures borderline for osteoporosis
- Needs to decrease weight, improve muscle tone, balance, and stability

- Needs to reduce belly fat and lower her BMI

Sally is a fun and energetic woman who loves friends and social gatherings. She always hated gyms and exercising. However, she was propelled into thinking about fitness when she unexpectedly divorced and wanted to start dating. She scheduled an appointment with a weight-loss doctor and had a physical exam prior to cosmetic surgery for a facelift.

Both doctors told her the same thing: if she didn't change her lifestyle, no matter how young her face looked or how much weight she lost, she was at high risk for heart disease and diabetes. Furthermore, she'd lost bone density and any fall would probably result in fractures.

Working with a wellness coach, she identified two activities that she enjoyed: walks with friends and dancing. She joined a local weight-loss group where she could socialize with new friends. After two months, she agreed to reconsider an exercise program at a gym.

Eventually, she found a group of friends to go to the gym with, started working with a trainer, and then augmented her gym routine with two days a week of walking one mile at a normal pace. She began tango lessons and went dancing with a weekly senior singles group.

Sally discovered that a Mediterranean diet, which allowed her to "cheat" one day per week, worked well for her. During the first year, Sally increased her walks to two miles, twice a week. She still didn't like the gym and eventually dropped out. She replaced it with a senior Zumba class, which gave her great cardio exercise and helped with weight loss.

After one full year, due to her dedication, Sally's BMI dropped to 21.1, and she lowered her weight from 160 to 135. Her risk for obesity and diabetes dropped into the safe zones. Sally acquired much better balance through dancing, and is careful about not falling.

Her cosmetic surgery was a success. She recently met someone online, then had several in-person dates and decided to play the field for a while. She says she now has confidence in herself, both inside and out, and feels for the first time like she's in charge of her health.

Sally changed her life.

Case Study: Roger

- Roger T., a 71-year-old male, weight 168, and height 6' 1", with a BMI of 22.2 (normal)
- Chronic fatigue
- Generally low vitality

- Forgetfulness
- Medication side effects
- Diminished appetite and recent weight loss
- Depression
- Had not exercised in 25 years

We connected Roger with two fitness partners. One walked with Roger three mornings a week, beginning with one mile. The other partner accompanied Roger to yoga class one day per week and meditation sessions two days a week.

After six months, Roger joined a gym and began body weight training two days per week. His walks turned into power walks and he increased his distance to four miles, three days per week.

Roger changed his diet to meals that included "real foods" high in nutrients and antioxidants.

After one year, Roger's fatigue and depression disappeared, his appetite returned, and he gained 15 pounds of muscle, while his body fat percentage dropped to 18.9.

Roger's appearance was deceptive. He had given the impression of a tall, lean, healthy man, when all the while he was decaying inside. When he told us about his chronic fatigue and loss of appetite, we began to probe into his level of fitness. When we learned there was none, we counseled him toward changing his life through walking, yoga, and meditation. Once he felt better about himself, it was relatively easy to get him to alter his diet and begin resistance workouts. Today Roger has completely overcome his enduring fatigue and his forgetfulness.

Case Study: Leo

- Leonardo L., a 68-year-old male, weight 215 and height 5' 8", BMI 32.7 (obese)
- Stomach ulcers
- Diverticulosis (small pockets in the wall of colon)
- Colon inflammation or colitis from infection or ischemia (poor blood flow)
- Swallowing difficulty (dysphasia)
- Constipation, bowel incontinence, and hemorrhoids

Leo was a gastrointestinal poster boy, and even though he could barely digest a meal, he was dangerously overweight and overate regularly. Leo didn't feel comfortable in a gym or on a track. He had been a high school tennis player and decided to revisit the sport. This "fun" activity began with one session a week with a hitting coach.

He focused on his diet by dropping processed foods and sugar and concentrating on fiber, fruits, and vegetables. After six weeks, he increased his tennis lessons to three days a week, and after six months he felt healthy enough to join a gym, hire a trainer, and begin light weight resistance and machine training.

After one year, Leo's ulcers, diverticulosis, and inflammation were under control and his other gastrointestinal issues were gone. Today Leo is not only symptom-free but he is also medication-free. His weight dropped to under 200 pounds and his BMI is in the safe zone.

Barry's Story

A few years back, my friend Barry decided to join me at the gym a few weeks after celebrating his 50th birthday. Barry was a big, healthy, strong hulk who had been sedentary for several years. Turning 50 influenced his subconscious mind, nagging him to do something, realizing that he was getting older. Barry was unwed and searching for his soul mate.

Even though I am some 20 years Barry's senior, I recommended to him that on his first day out he should take it easy and not attempt to lift as much weight or keep up with my pace.

Unfortunately, that advice went unheeded once we got started in the gym. Barry's competitive juices kicked in; he wanted to prove that he was a "real man." He willed his body to maintain the same pace along with the same weight load as this "senior man." On numerous occasions I admonished Barry to slow down and not chance an injury—after all, I had been doing this for years.

To prove his virility, Barry pushed and strained his way through our entire workout. The result was that Barry didn't set foot in that gym for six months, and when he did he refused to work out with me. I lost a good friend and a workout buddy due to some ego-filled male adrenaline rush.

As I told Barry, know in advance that there will be some soreness. This soreness is like falling off a bike; you must get back up, and in our case, back in the gym, to work through mild discomfort. The good news is that when you do the same activity again, your muscles will respond and quickly start to get used to it. You should have no soreness or less soreness because now you've strengthened the muscles and connective tissue. And this can happen quickly, if you are consistent and regularly use each muscle group.

Case Study: Rory

- Rory D., a 63-year-old male, weight 175 and height 5' 6" with a BMI of 31.5 (obese)
- Chronic obstructive pulmonary disease

- Loss of lung volume
- Shortness of breath
- Difficulty sleeping

Rory was a lifelong smoker and had been suffering the damage tobacco had ravaged on his lungs for years. We started him on a walking program (the first day he could only manage 100 yards). Patsi used hypnotherapy to wean him off his tobacco addiction.

After one month, Rory was walking one mile and had quit smoking. He hydrated himself with six to eight (eight-ounce) glasses of non-caffeinated beverages per day. He was placed on a salt-free balanced diet with emphasis on low-fat protein foods, whole grains, and fresh fruits and vegetables.

After one year he stopped taking his diuretic medication, joined a gym, and lowered his BMI to a heart-healthy 24.9. His lung capacity has returned and he is power-walking three to five miles a day, four days a week. Best of all, Rory is 100 percent tobacco-free.

Case Study: Frank

- Frank K., 42-year-old male, weight 193 and height 5' 8" with a BMI of 29.3 (overweight)

- Congestive heart failure
- Irregular heart rhythm (atrial fibrillation)
- High blood pressure (hypertension)
- Atherosclerosis (hardening and narrowing of blood vessels)
- Peripheral artery disease

Frank was very young (42) when he suffered his first heart attack. He had been a Type A workaholic who indulged in the good life and loved his wine and after-dinner cigar.

Following his major heart episode, he joined the local YMCA and they offered a class known as "The Comeback Squad." Frank went every Monday and Friday and I joined him once for an hour of unbelievably light resistance training and an unchallenging cardio workout.

Frank died three years later.

Unfortunately, not all our case histories have Hollywood endings. Frank was an example of someone having a serious disease who tiptoed around recovery. I believe he never got enough activity to strengthen his heart. I could be wrong, of course, as I don't know his complete medical history, but I've seen this happen with other people following a health crisis. For their remaining years they are fearful of the potential damage that exercise might do to their condition... so they tiptoe through life and let everything decay.

If your exercise program is too light, if you're not stressing your muscles more than what you would be doing in tasks of daily living, you're not strengthening anything. Naturally, every case is different and you should seek your physician's knowledge and advice before beginning any exercise program.

Case Study: William

- William Q., a 70-year-old male, weight 265 and height 6' 5" with a BMI of 31.4 (obese)
- Osteoarthritis (inflammation of joints due to wear and tear)
- Osteoporosis (bone loss)
- Gout
- Belly fat

Big Bill was a former collegiate athlete who survived the high life of alcohol, rich foods, tobacco, and recreational drugs of his youth. Bill began suffering debilitating joint pain in his late 50s. Twenty years later he existed on ibuprofen and prescription pain killers. When we met Bill, he was walking with a cane and was addicted to opiates.

Initially Bill changed his diet to feature omega-3 fatty acids, calcium, magnesium, ginger, and cayenne pepper, which depletes the pain-signaling chemical substance P. Bill's high levels of body fat helped him float in his pool and he actively started to swim, 15 to 25 minutes, five days a week.

After six months, Bill chucked his cane and joined our gym. He spent most of his time on low impact cardio machines and eventually began weight training twice a week.

Today Bill still suffers from osteoarthritis but no longer requires pain meds. His gout has been in remission for three years and he has lost 42 pounds.

Case Study: Carl

- Carl P., a 73-year-old male, weight 181 and height 5' 11" and a BMI of 25.2 (overweight)
- Prostate cancer
- Otherwise good health

Carl was diagnosed early with stage I prostate cancer at age 73 and was treated with hormonal therapy. During therapy, he altered his diet to include at least one-third raw food, increased animal-based omega-3 fats, eliminated sugars and processed foods, and added natural probiotics to reduce inflammation and strengthen his immune system response.

On the advice of his oncologist, Carl joined a gym and did cardio and weight training three days a week because his doctor explained that exercise lowers insulin levels, creating a low sugar environment to discourage the growth of cancer cells.

Today Carl is in remission. He tells us that due to his new diet and fitness regimen, he feels healthier and happier than ever.

Case Study: Lowell

- Lowell V., a 55-year-old male, height 6' and weight 170 with a BMI of 23.6 (normal)
- Medicine-induced insomnia
- Sleep deprivation
- Stress
- Frequent urination (benign prostatic hyperplasia, BPH, is an enlarged prostate)
- Arthritis

The older Lowell got, the more prominent his sleep problems became. He fought to stay up later to tire himself sufficiently to get to sleep and remain asleep throughout the night. Lowell reported, "I'm sleepy all the time; I go out at night and I fall asleep at the movies."

Lowell began to exercise three days per week at a gym. He did the treadmill and light free weights. He also took a beginning yoga class one day a week and swam for 15 minutes on Saturdays and Sundays.

Lowell's biggest change came in his diet. He ate a mix of protein and carbs for breakfast, and grazed at six 250-calorie mini meals throughout the day. He found that eating something nutritious every few hours helped his body and brain maintain the right balance of hormones and neurotransmitters, essential for falling and staying asleep at night.

Today Lowell is healthy and more energetic. He gets to sleep early and wakes early, but his sleep is deep and virtually uninterrupted. His stress is under control due to his exercise routine and his insomnia is gone due to his much-improved diet.

Case Study: Paul

- Paul W., a 63-year-old male, height 5' 10" and weight 154 with a BMI of 22.8 (normal)
- Forgetfulness, disorganization, confusion
- Neck ache, back pain, muscle spasms
- Nervous habits, fidgeting, feet tapping
- Difficulty concentrating, racing thoughts

- Depression, frequent or wild mood swings

During an interview with Patsi, it became clear that Paul has behavioral, physical, cognitive, and emotional symptoms of stress and anxiety. He had recently bought a house and was volunteering with several charities. Paul had volunteered to manage finances for one of his charities, and even though he was retired, his level of stress was enormous. Paul also led a very sedentary life and ate out often.

Meditation, yoga, and walking were suggested but Paul quickly rejected them. Next, he tried hiking, biking, and tennis with the same negative results. Paul found that he loved water aerobics and made that his four-times-a-week passion.

Paul began a regimen of water for hydration, calming teas and low-glycemic-index foods that released energy into his body at a slower, steady rate, allowing his body to process energy efficiently. His diet consisted of mostly nuts & berries, legumes, most vegetables, fruits, wheat grass and alfalfa. Paul also supplemented his diet with omega-3 fatty acids.

Today, all of Paul's symptoms have either vanished or are under his control. Like Paul, there are many seniors experiencing emotional and physical disorders that have been linked to stress. These include depression, anxiety, heart attacks, stroke, hypertension, immune system disturbances that increase susceptibility to infections, a host of viral - inked disorders ranging from the common cold to certain cancers, as well as autoimmune diseases like rheumatoid arthritis and allergies.

Case Study: Marco

- Marco S., a 65-year-old male, weight 173 and height 5' 10" with a BMI of 25.8 (normal)
- Early onset dementia
- Depression
- Weakened immune system
- Diminished sense of taste and smell

Marco had lost much of his taste and smell senses due to heavy smoking in his middle years. He began his comeback by running on weekends and pushed too hard. He switched to mountain biking until he fell and quit. He joined a gym and lasted only a few weeks. Marco finally discovered volleyball and jumped into it with a passion.

Marco modified his diet and became one of the few people I know to adopt a calorie reduction regimen of two meals per day—skipping dinner. After one year, he set up his home gym and added body resistance training three times a week.

Marco claims that his depression is gone and his dementia has improved. His BMI is now below 20 and his waistline has narrowed by four inches.

Marco is one of our most interesting senior cases. He appeared to be healthy but he was terribly depressed. He was already very active but could not maintain his interest in any activity. Very few people buy into the reduced-calorie diet concept, and maybe because Marco had lost much of his passion for food, he had little or no problem dropping one-third of his daily calorie intake. Today Marco claims that he is seldom sick and that some of his taste senses have returned, but most importantly, he is no longer suffering from depression.

Case Study: Carlos

- Carlos P., a 58- year- old male, height 5' 8" and weight 248 with a BMI of 37.7 (obese)
- Extra belly fat around the waist
- Low self-esteem
- Breathlessness
- Increased sweating
- Snoring
- Difficulty sleeping
- Inability to cope with physical activity
- Feeling very tired every day

- Back and joint pain (osteoarthritis)

Carlos had been overweight since his teens, but recently obesity had crept up on him without his even noticing. He was worried about more serious complications such as heart disease and stroke, and he had tried some radical diets which did little to abate continual weight gain.

Carlos started walking just two to five minutes per day, and then added an extra two minutes every third day. His initial goal was to walk 30 minutes per day. Riding a stationary bike was the next form of low-impact exercise. For Carlos, a recumbent bike was much more comfortable than a standard cycling seat. He began with five minutes, with a goal of fifteen.

After three months, Carlos' joint pain abated and his breathing improved enough to add fifteen minutes on the treadmill, along with the fifteen minutes on the recumbent bike. He added 20 minutes of water aerobics twice a week.

Carlos always hydrated with water due to the inordinate amount of sweat created by his workouts. After six weeks, Carlos had lost 12 lbs., which was just the beginning. His diet consisted of a complex-carb regimen, which he consumed only when he was hungry. He stopped drinking beer, caffeine, and sodas.

After six months, Carlos had dropped 28 pounds. He was no longer breathless or tired all day. His self-esteem allowed him to go shirtless at the pool for the first time in years.

After one year Carlos dropped out of the obese category and below 30.0 BMI. His back and joint pain disappeared and his weight dipped below 200 pounds.

Carlos' diet has had some starts and stops over the last five years; however, he has maintained his exercise regimen and even added resistance weight training. Due to his increased exercise, he has grown muscle and lost body fat. All nine of his previous obesity symptoms have disappeared. Today, at 63, Carlos has dramatically altered his health span.

When we look back at Carlos' results, he didn't begin to drop weight until he accepted and embraced his dietary transformation. And the biggest change was for him to spend the time to shop, read food labels, and select only "real food."

NOTES

Chapter 1

[1]   Ray Kurzweil and Terry Grossman, MD, <u>Transcend: Nine Steps to Living Well Forever</u> (New York: Rodale Inc., 2011), 15-17.

[2]   Ray Kurzweil and Terry Grossman, MD, <u>Transcend: Nine Steps to Living Well Forever</u> (New York: Rodale Inc., 2011), 47-50, 205-206.

[3]   Christiane Northrup, <u>Goddesses Never Age</u> (New York: Hay House Inc., 2015).

Chapter 2

[1]   Warburton et al, "<u>Health benefits of physical activity: the evidence</u>", *Canadian Medical Association Journal*, March 14, 2006.

Chapter 4

[1]   John C. Schell & Jared Rutter, <u>Mitochondria link metabolism and epigenetics in haematopoiesis</u>, *Nature Cell Biology* 19, 589-591.

[2]   Chris Crowley and Henry S. Lodge, <u>Younger Next Year: Live Strong, Fit and Sexy – Until You're 80 and Beyond</u> (New York: Workman Publishing).

Chapter 5

[1] "Deputy UN chief calls for urgent action to tackle global sanitation crisis," *UN News Centre,* March 21, 2013.

[2] "Lack of Sleep May Lead to Dementia: New Research Finds It Makes Brain Vulnerable," California Magazine, June 2, 2015.

Chapter 6

[1] "Environmental Toxins & Liver Disease: A Link?" WebMD, May 29, 2009.

[2] NIH, Overweight and Obesity Statistics.

[3] "Exercise", University of Maryland Medical Center, March 14, 2006.

[4] "Prevention and Risk of Alzheimer's and Dementia," Alzheimer's Association.

Chapter 7

[1] "Less Than 3 Percent of Americans Live a 'Healthy Lifestyle'," *The Atlantic,* March 23, 2016.

[2] "Belly fat in men: Why weight loss matters," Mayo Clinic, April 28, 2016.

Chapter 9

[1]   "Facts and Statistics," President's Council on Fitness, Sports and Nutrition, Dept. of Health and Human Services.

[2]   "Facts and Statistics," President's Council on Fitness, Sports and Nutrition, Dept. of Health and Human Services.

[3]   "You're Never Too Old: Keep Active as You Age," NIH News in Health, Dec. 2011.

Chapter 11

[1]   Daniel J. DeNoon, Weight Training for Heart Disease, *WebMD Medical News*, July 16, 2007.

[2]   Dr. Mercola, "Can You Really Get Fit in Six Minutes Per Week?", May 27, 2017.

Chapter 13

[1]   "Brisk Walk Healthier Than Running – Scientists", *The Guardian*, April 5, 2013.

Chapter 14

[1]   Thompson et al, "Does Participating in Physical Activity in Outdoor Natural Environments Have a Greater Effect on Physical and Mental Wellbeing Than Physical Activity Indoors? A Systematic Review", *Environmental Science & Technology*, February 3, 2011.

Chapter 16

1   Amy Capetta and Carey Rossi, "Being a Normal Weight With Extra Belly Fat Is Deadlier Than Being Obese," MSN.com, February 24, 2017.

2   Gretchen Reynolds, "Ask Well: Reducing Belly Fat," *New York Times*, May 15, 2015.

3   Erin Schumacher, "Pretty Much Nobody In The U.S. Leads A Healthy Lifestyle," *Huffpost*, March 25, 2016.

Appendix 1

1   Alzheimer's Disease Fact Sheet, National Institute on Aging.

2   Yaakov Stern PhD, "Cognitive Reserve in Ageing and Alzheimer's Disease," *The Lancet*, November 2012.

3   Michelle Trudeau, "Aerobic Exercise May Improve Memory in Seniors," NPR blog, February 21, 2011.

4   Erickson et al, "Exercise Training Increases Size of Hippocampus and Improves Memory," Proceedings of the National Academy of Sciences of the United States of America, vol. 108 no. 7.

5   Jason Selk, "Amidst Billion-Dollar Brain Fitness Industry, a Free Way to Train Your Brain," *Forbes*, August 13, 2013.

6   Ray Kurzweil and Terry Grossman, MD, Transcend: Nine Steps to Living Well Forever (New York: Rodale Inc., 2011).

Made in the USA
Middletown, DE
02 April 2019